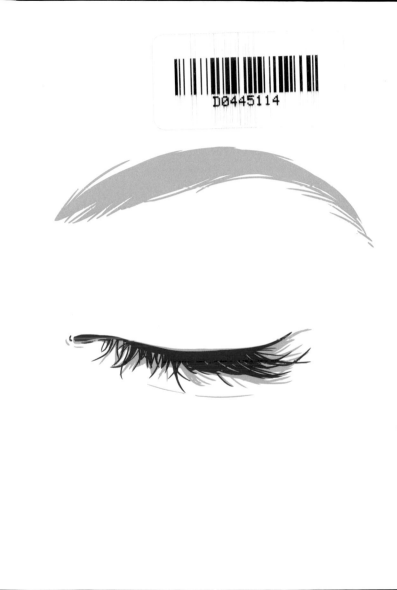

D0445114

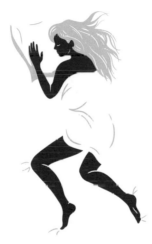

I want to sleep

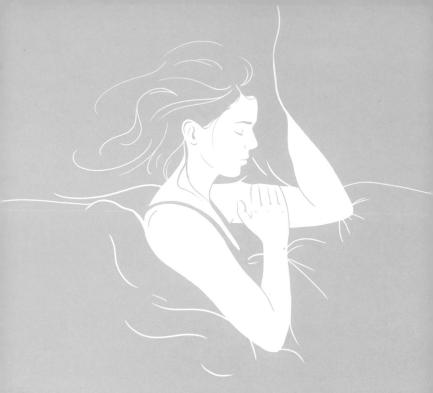

For Jane Johnson – I hope it helps.

Other books in the *I want to...* series:

I want to be calm

I want to sleep

HOW TO GET A GOOD NIGHT'S SLEEP

— BY —

Harriet Griffey

Contents

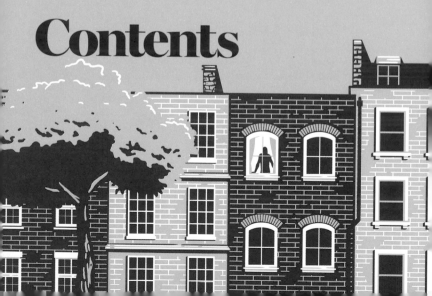

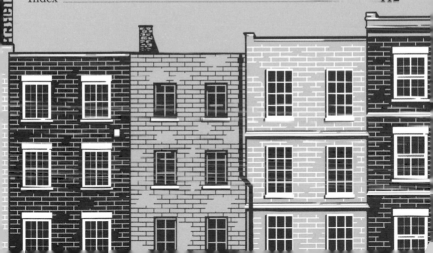

Part 2: How you can fix things

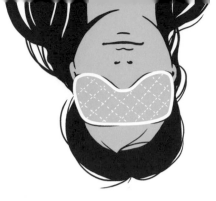

What is sleep?

Of all the body's functions, sleep is perhaps the most mysterious. We are unaware of most of what happens to us as we sleep and generally don't think about it, but given its importance to good health, sleep is one of the most important gifts we can give ourselves and one that any fairy godmother would wish to bestow on a child.

But when it goes wrong and we're not getting enough sleep, what can we do? Given the increasingly complex and busy lives we lead – far removed from our ancestors who, without the benefit of artificial light, functioned mainly during daylight hours and slept when it was dark – it is unsurprising that sleep can sometimes prove elusive or even impossible. We respond to all sorts of outside influences and psychological promptings that can keep us tense and alert and sleep at bay.

So why is sleep so important to our health? And what can you do to restore nourishing, peaceful sleep?

Nearly 6 in 10 adults in Britain – more than 28 million people – are sleep deprived and get 7 hours or less each night. This is a significant increase on the 2013 figure of 39 per cent. *Richard Wiseman, Professor in the Public Understanding of Psychology at the University of Hertfordshire*

But does being bleary-eyed by day matter? If this is because you are regularly getting less than six hours a night, then yes: it increases the risk of dying from heart disease by almost 50 per cent, and from stroke by 15 per cent according to a 2011 investigation carried out by Warwick University in the UK. Both conditions are associated with chronic inflammation of the cardiovascular system.

Anything you do to work against your body clock will have consequences on your physiology. *Francesco Cappuccio, Professor of Cardiovascular Medicine at Warwick*

When you're not getting enough sleep and are exhausted, it's sometimes hard to know how to fix things. The good news is that even small changes can make a big difference and, by following the steps in this book, you'll be able to get more sleep – and feel much better for it.

The last refuge of the insomniac is a sense of superiority to the sleeping world. *Leonard Cohen*

The following chapters will explain how sleep works so that you can begin to work out where and when in the 24-hour wake–sleep cycle things are going wrong – and what you can do to fix things.

Sleep is the best meditation.

DALAI LAMA

PART 1

The science bit

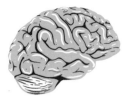

Why we sleep

Even if much of what happens to us when we sleep is a mystery to us; that it is restorative and we spend a third of our lives doing it suggests that sleep is crucial for mind and body. But thinking of it as a passive activity is a mistake. During that time of peaceful, apparent oblivion, there's a lot going on.

As I spent more time investigating the science of sleep, I began to understand that these strange hours of the night underpin every moment of our lives. *David K. Randall, author of* Dreamland: Adventures in the Strange Science of Sleep

Much of what we understand about the benefits of sleep comes from how we feel when we don't get enough of it. Mentally and physically lethargic, easily distracted, irritable and with slower reaction times – we just don't feel great when we don't sleep well. An occasional bad night won't matter much, but sleep deprivation is serious if we are attempting tasks that rely on us being alert and having good reaction times. Like driving a car. Dozing off at the wheel is a well-known cause of driving accidents, many of which have catastrophic and fatal results.

For drivers of all ages, estimates in the United States, United Kingdom and Australia report that between 5 and 30 per cent of crashes are attributed to fatigue. Not only are drivers more likely to have sleep-related crashes; these crashes are more likely to be fatal compared with other crash causes.
The George Institute for Global Health in Sydney, Australia, 2013

Sleep is essential for allowing the cortex of the brain – responsible for planning, decision-making and problem-solving – to take some time out. The cortex isn't completely inactive when we sleep, but it slows down, allowing space for the processing and consolidation of memory. When we have a problem to solve – mentally, emotionally and even physically – sleeping on it can sometimes yield good results.

It is a common experience that a problem difficult at night is resolved in the morning after the committee of sleep has worked on it. *John Steinbeck*

In a study carried out by Drs Fisher and Dement in the US in the 1950s, a group of volunteers were woken during dreaming sleep (REM sleep, see page 23) over five consecutive nights. They showed signs of tension, anxiety, difficulty in concentrating, irritability and a tendency to hallucinate. When allowed to sleep normally after this period, an increase in the amount of REM sleep occurred. There was no indication of any long-term damage following the experiment.

Sleep also rests our bodies, although that doesn't mean that energy isn't burnt. Sleep burns around 80 calories an hour, not far short of the 95 calories used when watching television.

Unsurprisingly, secretion of those hormones responsible for wakefulness – corticosteroids and adrenaline – is reduced by sleep. This inhibition of wakeful hormones allows the release of growth hormone by the pituitary gland, responsible not only for cell growth but also cell renewal, which occurs mainly during stage 3 and 4 sleep (see page 27). In growing children sleep takes on a special significance because of this, but it is still relevant for adults. After strenuous exercise, or during pregnancy, for example, sleep needs can increase.

Proven benefits of sleep

> Increases ability to concentrate and remember new information.
> Helps maintain a healthy weight.
> Reduces stress and improves mood.
> Improves athletic performance and coordination.

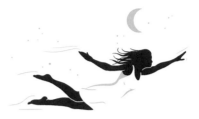

Functions of sleep

**Sleep, that knits up the ravell'd sleeve of care,
The depth of each day's life, sore labour's bath,
Balm of hurt minds, great nature's second course,
Chief nourisher in life's feast.** Macbeth (*Act 2, scene II*)

The main purpose of sleep is to rest both the body and mind, although it is the mind that is most immediately affected by sleep shortage. It is, however, insidious: the effects of low-grade chronic sleep deprivation creep up on us. A couple of poor nights of sleep and we can quickly recover, but over time it can affect not only our brain power but also our immune and cardiovascular systems. Sleep deprivation affects mood and concentration, causes aggression and forgetfulness, paranoia, hallucinations and confusion, along with blurred vision and slurred speech.

Sleep is needed for the body's nervous systems to work properly
Sleep gives brain cells a chance to repair themselves. Brain cells can become exhausted or so polluted with the process of normal cell activity that, without time out, they begin to malfunction. Sleep may also give unused brain cells an opportunity to connect, ensuring that they don't deteriorate from lack of activity.

Sleep, especially deep sleep, also allows a reduction of activity in those parts of the brain that control emotions, decision-making processes and social interactions. This may help people maintain good emotional and social relationships while they are awake – and is probably why, without sleep, we can get grumpy or aggressive.

Dreaming
Dreams occur during periods of REM sleep (see page 23) – whether or not you remember them when you wake. Many theories about the importance of dreams exist, from Freud to Jung. Some believe that the cortex, the part of the brain that interprets and organises information when we're awake, tries to interpret the random signals resulting from fragmented brain activity during REM sleep, producing the stories we experience as dreams.

We all dream. We do not understand our dreams, yet we act as if nothing strange goes on in our minds, strange at least by comparison with the logical, purposeful doings of our minds when we are awake.

ERICH FROMM

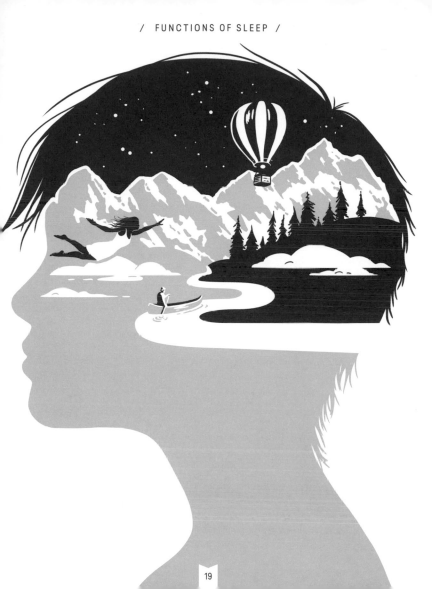

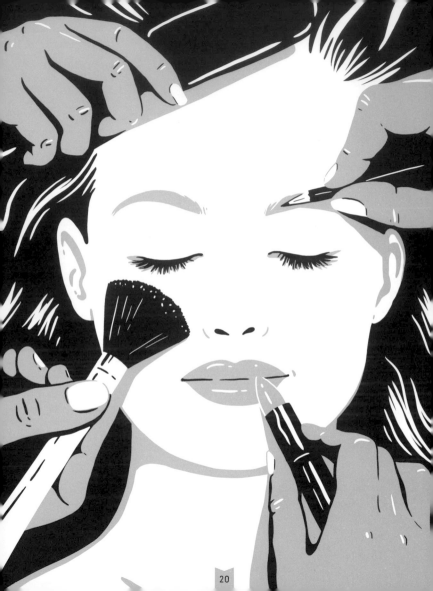

It's thought that this process also serves in some way to de-clutter or de-fragment the brain, creating new connections that we might resist while awake and that this can, in some way, allow emotional therapy. Hence the reasoning behind the benefit of sleeping on a problem: on waking, we seem to find solutions that eluded us before.

Dreams also stabilise our moods, as the processing of emotional memories also occurs during REM sleep. Without adequate REM sleep, we lose a valuable resource in our ability to manage our moods, which is why we can become 'tired and emotional' without it, something that's particularly easy to see in sleep-deprived children.

Beauty sleep

Deep sleep allows the release of growth hormone in children and young adults, with the body's cells showing increased activity, combined with the reduced breakdown of proteins during sleep. Proteins are the building blocks needed for cell growth and for repair of damage. In addition, stress hormones like cortisol, produced while awake and in response to sleep deprivation, inhibit the production of collagen, which we need to keep wrinkles at bay. Several periods of good, deep sleep a night (at least five 90-minute sleep cycles a night) will provide the beauty sleep we need.

Sleep is that golden chain that ties health and our bodies together. *Thomas Dekker*

The sleep–immune system connection

The neurons that control sleep interact closely with the immune system. When we are unwell, as anyone who has had the flu knows, infectious diseases tend to make us feel sleepy. This is because cytokines – the chemicals in our immune system produced when the body is fighting infection – make us sleepy. Sleep may also help the body conserve energy and the other resources that the immune system needs to tackle infection. This also means that a lack of sleep can lead to us being stressed and can lead to illness.

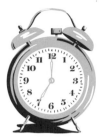

Sleep cycles

Although we may think of sleep as a time when we do nothing, in fact there's a lot going on in our minds and bodies. A series of stages take place that occur in cycles throughout the time we spend asleep.

A complete sleep cycle consists of four stages of what is called non-REM (Rapid Eye Movement) sleep and one of REM sleep, during which dreaming occurs. And while a baby's sleep cycle is around 50 minutes, by adulthood it's extended to around 90 minutes.

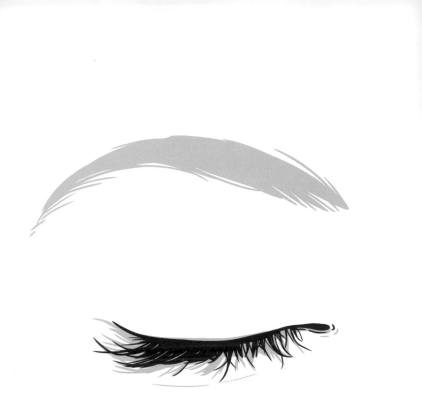

Sleep is no mean art: for its sake

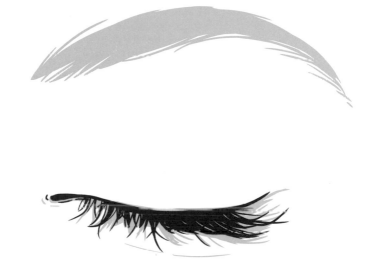

one must stay awake all day.

FRIEDRICH NIETZSCHE

Stages of the sleep cycle

> *Stage 1* non-REM sleep is when we move from full wakefulness to the drowsy precursor of sleep, when it's almost inevitable that we will drift off, but not quite. During this phase we are equally capable of either nodding off completely, or waking up instantly.

> *Stage 2* is a very definite, but light, sleep cycle, and it's during this phase that you might be susceptible to a 'hypnagogic startle' – when you are briefly jolted awake by a muscular jerk. Irritating though this can be, it serves no purpose and does no damage.

> *Stages 3 to 4* move you into deeper sleep, where it would be difficult to wake you, although you would respond to a baby's cry, an alarm or other sudden noise or having your name called. Breathing and heart rate are very regular, slow and stable. This is the phase of sleep that restores us physically the most.

> *An EEG* (electroencephalogram) trace of brain waves during these four stages would show quite definite changes. During stage 1, brain waves move from Alpha (alert) to Beta and into Theta activity, before moving into the recognisable Delta activity of deep sleep, where the EEG trace shows a pattern of deep, slow waves.

> *REM sleep* is a phase that occurs at the end of stage 4 non-REM sleep, before moving back to stage 1. An EEG would show distinct changes in brain waves, moving in and out of Theta and Beta activity during this more active, dreaming phase of sleep. Breathing and heart rate increases and rapid eye movement is clearly seen under the eyelids. Conversely, during this phase the body's muscles are in such deep relaxation it is almost akin to paralysis, and nerve impulses are effectively blocked to limit any movement that could arise from the internal activity of our dreams. If we wake, or are woken, during this phase we can experience a temporary feeling of being unable to move.

When it comes to sleep stages, cycles and patterns, the body has a self-regulating facility that is largely outside our control, although it can be affected and does respond to outside events. We can decide when to sleep or not, but not what patterns emerge when we do sleep. When there is a definite sleep deficit, however, and we need more deep sleep to

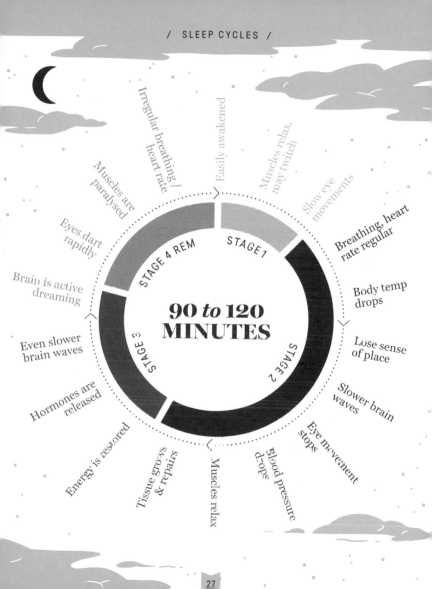

STAGE 1
STAGE 2
STAGE 3
STAGE 4 REM

90 to 120 MINUTES

Easily awakened
Irregular breathing/heart rate
Muscles are paralysed
Eyes dart rapidly
Brain is active dreaming
Even slower brain waves
Hormones are released
Energy is restored
Tissue grows & repairs
Muscles relax
Blood pressure drops
Eye movement stops
Slower brain waves
Lose sense of place
Body temp drops
Breathing, heart rate regular
Slow eye movements
Muscles relax, may twitch

compensate, then the period of deep sleep is extended within the cycle. In addition, the longer and better we sleep, successive periods of REM sleep tend to become longer, but we have little control over that either.

What can affect an individual sleep pattern is the use of medication, not only over-the-counter herbal, antihistamine or prescription sleeping pills, but also recreational drugs like alcohol or cannabis. The effect on sleep stages, for example, moving you straight from stage one to stage four, can sometimes be helpful in the short term, but it does affect the cycle of sleep stages. While a small nightcap can be a relaxing bonus at the end of a busy day, using alcohol or other drugs to reach oblivion has a detrimental effect, changing the natural pattern of sleep and causing you to wake a few hours later.

Sleep patterns also change throughout our lives. The sleep pattern of a baby is very different to that of an adult, and an adolescent's pattern is different to that of an elderly person's (see pages 45–61).

How do people go to sleep? I'm afraid I've lost the knack. I might try busting myself smartly over the temple with the night-light. I might repeat to myself, slowly and soothingly, a list of quotations from minds profound; if I can remember any of the damn things.

DOROTHY PARKER

When should you wake up?

The 90-minute sleep cycle is repeated as we sleep and it's worth bearing this in mind when you set your alarm clock. If you want to wake feeling alert – i.e. at the end of a 90-minute cycle – it's a good idea to count backwards in 90-minute chunks to work out when it's best to go to sleep. So, if you set your alarm for 8 a.m. it would be best to fall asleep at 11 p.m., as theoretically you should be naturally 'surfacing' at 8 a.m.

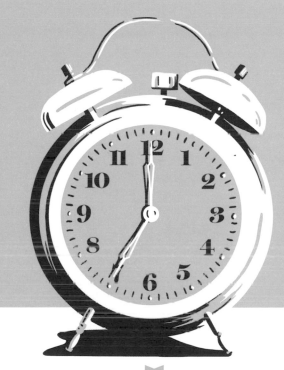

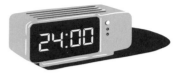

The 24-hour day

We are diurnal mammals, designed to be awake during the day and asleep at night, and even though we fight it with our 24/7 lifestyles, when it comes to sleep, it's worth thinking about how the internal 'body clock' works.

Everyone has an internal body clock that decides when you feel wakeful or sleepy, active or tired, hungry or not and, in less obvious ways, our hormone secretions and body temperature.

Our body clocks are generated by the Suprachiasmatic Nuclei (SCN) in a part of the brain known as the hypothalamus. Light receptor cells in the eye respond to light and keep the SCN in tune with the day, stopping the secretion of the sleep hormone melatonin. Light is essential: the alternating light and darkness of day and night is what synchronises us to the 24-hour day.

In fact, our bodies run roughly to a 24.5-hour clock, but we rely on physical cues – the time we get up, the spacing of mealtimes, the response to dark and light, the patterns we impose on our days – to help us to stay on a 24-hour track.

Think in the morning. Act in the noon. Eat in the evening. Sleep at night.

WILLIAM BLAKE

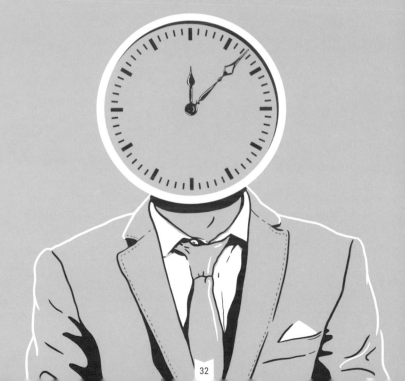

Body clock phases

 06:00 - TO - 09:00

Male testosterone peak. Highest incidence of heart attack. Melatonin production ceases – optimum time to wake. A poor time to exercise.

 09:00 - TO - 12:00

Stress hormone cortisol peaks. Maximum alertness – best time to work. Short-term memory at its best.

 12:00 - TO - 15:00

Increased gastric activity – either because you have just eaten or your body clock is telling you it's time to. Post-lunchtime dip in alertness. Peak time for road accident fatalities is at 14:00.

 15:00 - TO - 18:00

Core body temperature peaks. Best heart and lung capacity. Muscles are 6 per cent stronger than at other times. Best time for physical exercise.

 18:00 - TO - 21:00

Intuitive thinking is improved. Digestion of big meals is less effective. The liver, however, is more able to process alcohol than at lunchtime.

 21:00 - TO - 00:00

Dip in natural light stimulates melatonin production. Core body temperature drops. Optimum time for bed.

00:00 - TO - 03:00

Levels of melatonin peak. Bowels shut down for the night. Attention span at a minimum. Brain organises and consolidates memories.

03:00 - TO - 06:00

Core temperature low while body repair work occurs. Severe asthma attacks more common. Natural births tend to occur most.

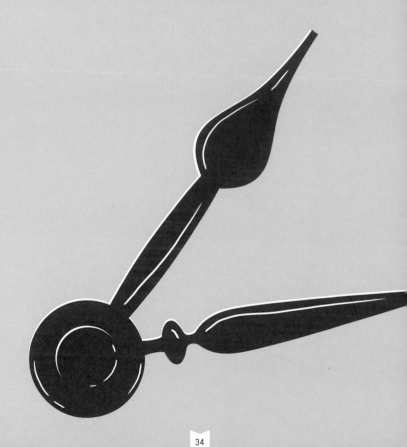

We are the supremely arrogant species; we feel we can abandon four billion years of evolution and ignore the fact that we have evolved under a light–dark cycle. What we do as a species, perhaps uniquely, is override the clock. And long-term acting against the clock can lead to serious health problems.

PROFESSOR RUSSELL FOSTER, UNIVERSITY OF OXFORD

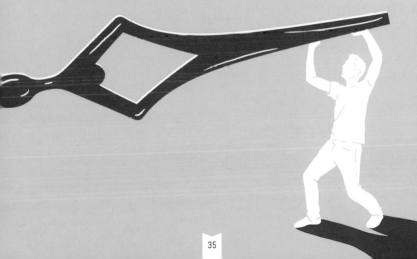

Out of sync

Having said all this, our circadian rhythms aren't written in stone; they are susceptible to external influences – jet lag, shift work or illness – that can create short- or long-term problems with sleep. This is caused by the timing of the release of two hormones: melatonin (from the pineal gland in the brain), which affects sleep and mood; and cortisol (from the adrenal glands), which is produced in response to stress or when blood sugar falls, and affects your metabolism, cardiovascular function, immune system and even your appetite. Because the release of melatonin and cortisol constantly fluctuates, even under normal circumstances, not every night's sleep will be the same. Sometimes you sleep well, another time less well, and poor sleep can happen when the mismatch of melatonin and cortisol put the body clock out of sync with the day–night cycle.

A lot of what we know about circadian rhythms and the 24-hour day comes from research on those who are not influenced by light – those who are blind, for example. We also know from those who are affected by Seasonal Affective Disorder (SAD) and who suffer from low mood and sleep problems, how important it is to be exposed to light each day.

Warning

Knowing the importance of being exposed to daylight every day, scientists have warned that modern life and our 24-hour society mean many people are now 'living against' their body clocks, with damaging consequences for their health and well-being.

When it comes to solving sleep problems, it's worth considering whether you help your 24-hour clock, or hinder it. Given that regular sleep is linked to the amount of light we are exposed to, it's worth taking a look at what is happening throughout the day, not just at night when you are trying to sleep.

ASK YOURSELF...

> Do you have regular times for waking and going to bed?
> Are you exposed to daylight, or full-spectrum lighting, for at least part of the day?
> If you take exercise each day, is this in the morning, afternoon or evening?
> Do you have a period of relaxing in less-bright light before going to bed?
> Is your bedroom dark at night?

We are creatures of habit and, much as young children respond to a regular lifestyle, so we do, too. That's not to say that we can't be flexible, or change things – for those working 9–5, Monday to Friday, most weekends are a change in schedule – we can adapt and, even if it means maybe a night or two of less good sleep, we can adjust. But sometimes, for a variety of reasons and in spite of our best efforts, we can hit a period of insomnia or early morning waking and need to review our lifestyle to get back on track. Chronic problems usually arise when – often for reasons of over-tiredness caused by other reasons – our body clock becomes completely skewed; the more tired we become, the more difficult it is to get back to sleeping well.

So that's when a look at your 24-hour day is a good first step towards better sleep.

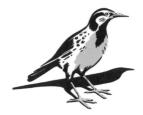

Lark or owl?

Are you, as the saying goes, a lark or an owl? Do you function best in the morning or late at night?

While society might be programmed for us to function best between 9–5, some of us really do struggle with this and it comes down to our genes, according to neurogeneticist Dr Louis Ptacek at the University of California, San Francisco, who is studying families that show evidence of Advanced Sleep Phase Syndrome (larks) and Delayed Sleep Phase Syndrome (owls). But the good news is, given that life today is much more 24/7, if we know which we are, we can work with this.

Are you a lark or an owl?

> If you usually have to get up at a specific time each day, how much do you depend on an alarm clock?

Every time – I can't wake up without one! *1 point*
Usually *2 points*
Sometimes *3 points*
Never *4 points*

> How hungry do you feel the first half hour after you wake up?

Ravenous *4 points*
Something light is good *3 points*
Sometimes hungry *2 points*
I never eat breakfast *1 point*

> Do you consider yourself to be a lark or an owl?

Possibly a morning type *3 points*
Possibly an evening type *2 points*
Definitely a morning type *4 points*
Definitely an evening type *1 point*

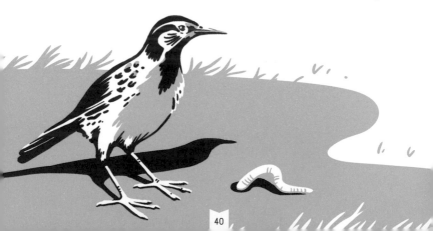

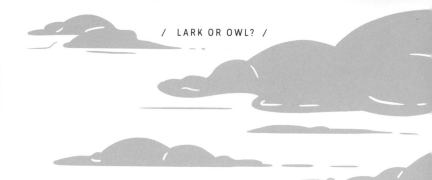

› If you had no commitments the next day, how much later than your usual bedtime would you go to bed?

No later – the same time .... *3 points*
An hour or two later .... *2 points*
I'd be up all night! .... *1 point*

› If you went to bed several hours later than normal, but there is no need to get up at a particular time the next morning, which is most likely to occur?

I'd wake the same time as usual .... *4 points*
I'd wake the same time but doze .... *3 points*
I'd wake at the usual time but fall back to sleep .... *2 points*
I wouldn't wake until much later than usual .... *1 point*

› You have to do two hours of physically hard work, in which of the following periods would you choose to do this?

08:00–10:00 .... *4 points*
12:00–14:00 .... *3 points*
15:00–17:00 .... *2 points*
19:00–21:00 .... *1 point*

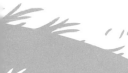

› You have a two-hour written exam to take, in which of the following periods would you choose to do this?

08:00–10:00	*4 points*
12:00–14:00	*3 points*
15:00–17:00	*2 points*
19:00–21:00	*1 point*

› A friend asks you to join him twice a week for a workout in the gym and the best time for him is between 22:00–23:00. How do you think you would perform?

Very well	*1 point*
OK	*2 points*
Poorly	*3 points*
I wouldn't do it!	*4 points*

› If you were free to plan your evening and had no commitments the next day, what time would you choose to go to bed?

21:00–22:00	*4 points*
22:00–23:00	*3 points*
23:00–00:00	*2 points*
00:00–01:00	*1 point*

Add up your score

35-30 POINTS	29-26 POINTS	25-20 POINTS	19-15 POINTS	14-9 POINTS
definitely a morning person	moderately a morning person	neither one nor the other	moderately an evening person	definitely an evening person

While being a lark or an owl may be genetically determined, we are also affected by our circadian rhythms. Sometimes known as our 'biological clock', these rhythms are influenced by the dark–light cycles of the 24-hour day and are regulated by the secretion of melatonin from the pineal gland in the brain in response to the amount of light received via the eye.

Of course while there is a great deal of difference between individuals, it is true to say that we are affected by light and that, while the invention of artificial light can sometimes be to our advantage, it can also work against our natural sleep patterns.

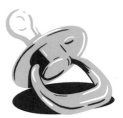

Babies & children

There never was a child so lovely but his mother was glad to see him sleep. *Ralph Waldo Emerson*

Chances are, if you have picked up this book and turned to this section first, you're a new parent – and probably not getting as much sleep as you'd like!

Newborn babies haven't got a clue about day or night and although they will spend most of their first few weeks virtually asleep all the time, with periods of wakefulness in between, they are already beginning to learn about day and night from what's going on around them, and alternating periods of light and dark can kick-start their hormonal regulators.

Along with light and dark, food is also one of the first cues for a baby, although in the early weeks when feeding routines are being established – especially breastfeeding – everything seems topsy-turvy. Once solids are

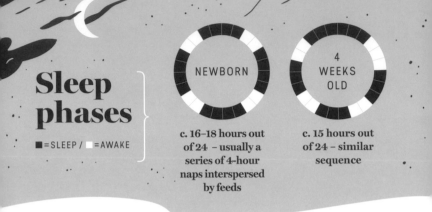

Sleep phases

■ = SLEEP / □ = AWAKE

NEWBORN

c. 16–18 hours out of 24 – usually a series of 4-hour naps interspersed by feeds

4 WEEKS OLD

c. 15 hours out of 24 – similar sequence

introduced at about six months, the introduction of more calorie-dense foods eaten during the day means that it is possible to drop the night-time milk feeds – this is important, because feeding at night can actually cause waking, both in anticipation of a feed and also because of having to digest it. Think about it: few of us would welcome a cheese sandwich at 3 a.m.

When a baby's more alert, wakeful times increase during the day by the scheduling of daytime activities; periods of being awake and being asleep can be nudged towards more sleep at night.

Sleep cycles in babies and children are shorter than in adults, too – around 50 to our 90-minute cycle – but they tend to hit deep sleep almost immediately upon falling asleep. This 50-minute cycle also means they will hit lighter sleep and 'surface' around once an hour.

Learning how to go to sleep

The trick to getting more sleep as a parent of a baby is to enable babies to learn to go back to sleep on their own, without needing a parent to help them. This means actively allowing a baby to learn to fall asleep on its

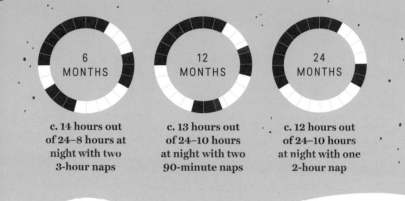

c. 14 hours out of 24–8 hours at night with two 3-hour naps

c. 13 hours out of 24–10 hours at night with two 90-minute naps

c. 12 hours out of 24–10 hours at night with one 2-hour nap

own; putting it down for its daytime nap before it has fully zonked out is a first start.

If a baby falls asleep in your arms mid-feed, or is rocked to sleep, it means that these circumstances – which are dependent on you – have to be replicated in order to be able to go to sleep again when waking at night. Often, what we do with hard-to-settle babies is feed them to sleep ... which is fine until they are six months old and still waking at 3 a.m. The other temptation is, on any sign of waking, leaping to attention and picking up the baby so it doesn't cry; this doesn't allow the baby to learn to go to sleep alone either. Introducing new routines is easier on everyone if done during the day, but make sure the room in which your baby sleeps is darkened.

Co-sleeping is a matter of choice for many parents, and works well for some, although it may make it more difficult for an older child to sleep alone beyond babyhood. But for most of us, having a baby sleep through the night is the objective; it makes family life easier for everyone in the long run. Helping a baby learn to go to sleep on his or her own – without another's physical presence – is the key to a baby sleeping through the night.

Over-tired?

Often parents will say: 'My baby doesn't need much sleep', but it's worth remembering that being over-tired stimulates both the cortisol and adrenaline (awake) hormones, which makes it harder for a baby or small child to settle. All that hyperactive behaviour might actually be a result of sleep deprivation and babies that are grizzly and fretful when awake are often exhausted and find it more difficult to settle in what is, effectively, a stressed state.

In this instance, maintaining a schedule for a while can help your baby become more flexible, rather than less so, as adaptation to anything is always easier if we've had enough sleep.

People who say they sleep like a baby usually don't have one.

LEO J. BURKE

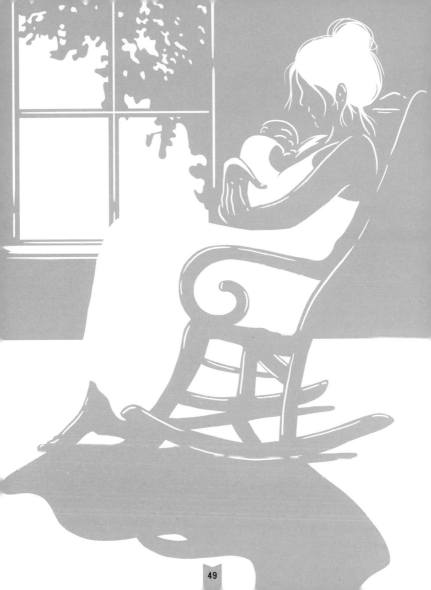

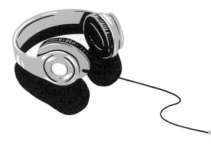

Teenagers

The scenario of the teenager burning the midnight oil and sleeping until noon is all too common, but it is rooted in the physical changes experienced during the transition from child to adult, and over which they have no control. The increased demands of physical growth and the re-organisation of the brain, combined with the impact of hormonal surges, all create a hyper-stimulated mix in the teenager.

Sleep deprivation

This is exacerbated by a 'sleep phase delay' that means the teenagers normal sleep pattern veers towards going to sleep later and, as a consequence, waking up later. The problem with falling asleep at 1 a.m. and then having to get up for school at 7 a.m. means an inevitable sleep deficit. As a result, and this will come as no surprise to their parents, chronic sleep deprivation is a common problem among teenagers, with some studies suggesting that up to 75 per cent will have problems.

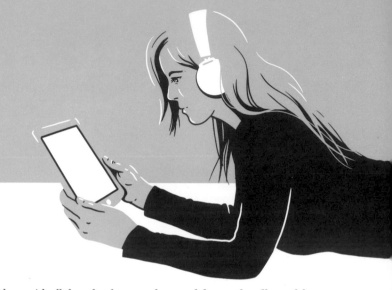

Along with all the other hormonal ups and downs, the effects of sleep deprivation can add to this toxic mix. Just a two-hour sleep deficit can have a marked effect on mood and attention span, while studies have shown a link to obesity and depression in the longer term; and in the short term an increase in colds, flu and gastroenteritis when teenagers get less sleep than they need.

Smartphones, laptops and computer games often encourage late nights, but the blue light they emit creates wakefulness by inhibiting the secretion of the sleep hormone melatonin. Using laptops in bed, texting and even reading from a Kindle may all contribute to this.

Given that an ideal amount of sleep for teenagers is nine hours, the consequences of this chronic sleep deprivation can make them tired, irritable, impatient and depressed. They don't just fall asleep in class, they often spend most of their weekends in bed, sleeping until midday, so they are effectively suffering from something akin to chronic jet lag.

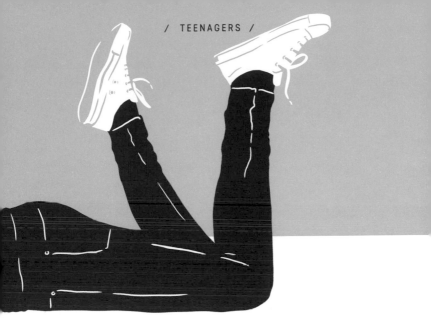

A study published in the US *Journal of Developmental and Behavioral Pediatrics* found that a 25-minute delay to the start of the school day improved the sleep patterns and mood of teenagers. It showed that if school schedules were more closely aligned with teenagers' circadian rhythms and sleep needs, students were more alert, happier, better prepared to learn, and not dependent on coffee and energy drinks just to stay awake in class. Daytime sleepiness, depressed mood and caffeine use were all significantly reduced after the later start time.

Over-tired or ADHD?

Experts have found that the symptoms of sleep deprivation and hyperactivity are similar, with some young people being diagnosed as having Attention Deficit Hyperactivity Disorder (ADHD) or even Asperger's. By instilling better sleep patterns and encouraging adequate sleep, symptoms of ADHD sometimes disappeared and many young people found that their ability to concentrate in school was improved.

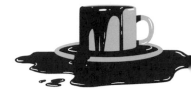

Adults

By the time we reach the age of 25, the hormonal tumult of the teenage years should have settled down, allowing us to get our sleep back on track and to fit in with the more routine 9–5 of working life.

There are certainly individual differences in the amount of sleep that people need. The acid test is whether you are sleepy throughout the next day or whether you are alert. Some people kid themselves that they can get by on little sleep, but in fact they have to nap during the afternoon to make up. *Professor Jim Horne*

Sleep cycles in adults are based on a 90-minute cycle and our sleep habits have become established. Some of us have been good sleepers from infancy, with seldom a care in the world to trouble our nights, while others are fitful, light sleepers with intermittent bouts of insomnia. However we sleep, only a few of us are getting as much as we probably need.

There is a time for words and there is also a time for sleep.
Homer

Our adult years can also be our most stressful. Although physical energy might be high and our mental prowess at its supposed peak, combining a demanding job with a social life or, in time, a young family brings its own pressures, and this can affect our sleep. For some, the demands of adult life may be the first time they encounter a sleep problem and the need to re-evaluate some of their habits. Where that one cup of coffee a day has become six, the long-hours culture of the working day has put paid to any regular exercise and the early morning waking has become the only way to catch up on basic chores: it's hard to cram it all in and sleep has become relegated to a short six or seven hours a night.

I'm always without sleep. I've got two kids. I understand sleep deprivation on a profound level.

CATE BLANCHETT

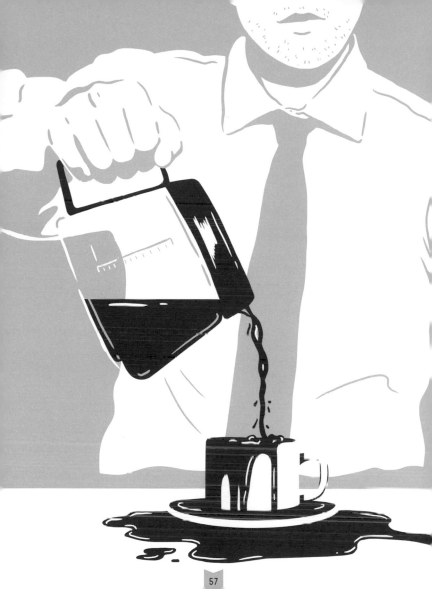

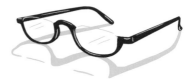

Older people

As we age, both our lifestyle and our physical need for sleep changes. Even if we sleep for the same length of time, sleep is lighter as there is not the same need for the deep, slow-wave sleep required by the growing body of a child or teenager.

Men and women tend to experience sleep problems differently, with women tending to suffer more from insomnia.

Men

Men may find that prostate enlargement makes more frequent urination a problem, not only for them but for their partner. Managing this may include restricting fluid intake for a couple of hours before bedtime, or bladder retraining (over-riding the sensation of wanting to go and getting the bladder used to holding more fluid before reaching this point) during the day. These can both help to avoid this problem during the night.

Women

Women tend to have more problems with sleep than men, and during menopause can be disturbed by symptoms of increased wakefulness that may be caused by 'night sweats'. Although laboratory-based research into this suggests that the beginnings of wakening actually preceded this and may be linked to the hormonal changes affecting the body clock, rather than the symptoms. Hormone replacement therapy can go a long way to easing menopausal symptoms for some, but alternative recommendations include the taking of a supplement of vitamin E, selenium and vitamin C with bioflavonoids to help alleviate symptoms, and following the advice given later in the book about good sleep practice (see page 95).

In the elderly...

Less physical activity, less daytime exposure to light, along with reduced intellectual stimulation and encroaching boredom, combined with too much daytime napping can all contribute to disrupted and poor night-time sleep.

Age-related illness like arthritis, which causes pain, can also create problems when trying to get comfortable enough to sleep peacefully. Cognitive disorders like dementia, where daytime confusion is also common, affect circadian rhythms and, consequently, night-time sleep. These sleep problems may arise from changes in the brain regions and neurotransmitters that control sleep, or from the drugs used to control symptoms of other disorders. Overmedication, too, can be a problem – excessive painkillers or night-time medication, for example – and can contribute, as the body tries to self-regulate its body clock.

Managing sleep problems in the elderly means re-establishing the rhythms of a 24-hour day, enabling the body clock to run most closely to a day–night schedule, and dealing with any external factors – pain, hunger, infection – that may be contributing to sleeplessness.

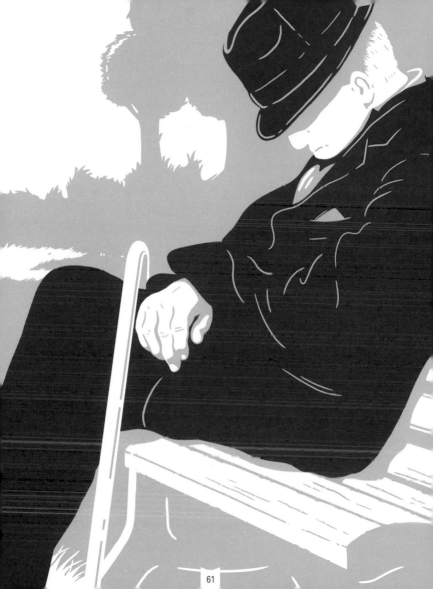

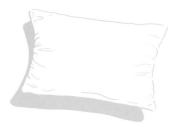

Sleep needs

A well-spent day brings happy sleep. *Leonardo da Vinci*

Although everyone varies in the amount of sleep that they need, and this changes with age, there is a general rule of thumb that suggests the basic amount of good, restorative sleep that we each need to feel and perform at our best.

Sleep needs through life

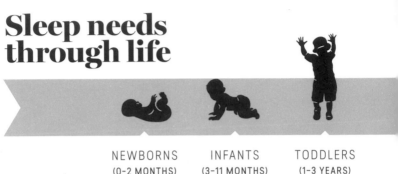

NEWBORNS	INFANTS	TODDLERS
(0-2 MONTHS)	(3-11 MONTHS)	(1-3 YEARS)
15–18 hours over	**14–15 hours over**	**12–14 hours**
a 24-hour period	**a 24-hour period**	**(mostly at night)**

What requires balance is the amount of sleep your body needs on a regular basis to feel good and perform well – known as your basal sleep need – and any sleep debt. Sleep debt is sleep lost over a period of one or several nights because of poor sleep habits, sickness, being woken by noise or other disturbances and other causes. When basal sleep need and sleep debt are out of balance, difficulty waking in the morning and general alertness and daytime sleepiness is experienced to a greater or lesser degree.

You may be suffering from a sleep deficit if:
› You find it difficult to wake each morning and feel groggy when you do.
› You are woken a couple of times a night by external noise or other disturbance.
› You find it difficult to concentrate for extended periods of time.
› You have not so much an 'energy dip' in the early afternoon, as an almost overwhelming desire to go to sleep.

Some people cope better with sleep debt than others. Some people find that sleep deficiency makes them feel unwell or unable to cope, which can

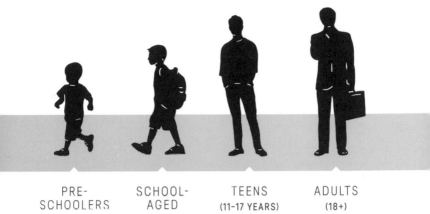

PRE-SCHOOLERS (3–5 YEARS)	SCHOOL-AGED (5–10 YEARS)	TEENS (11–17 YEARS)	ADULTS (18+)
11–13 hours	10–11 hours	8½–9½ hours	7–9 hours

lead to anxiety about managing the day's events or sleeping itself. Others just accept that they feel a little off, but expect to catch up on sleep and feel better because of it. In fact, we cope quite well with occasional sleep deficiency as long as we compensate for it in time with additional sleep.

When there is a psyche-disrupting event in your life, it can prevent you getting the long blocks of sleep at night that are so important to healthy aging. *Dr Mehmet Öz*

Some manage on far less sleep than the average. Margaret Thatcher, Mussolini, Mao Tse-tung and Hitler are examples of the five per cent of the population that could happily (although we might query that with the examples above!) manage on only three to four hours' sleep a night.

But if you are someone who feels they are continually sleep deprived, it's worth looking into the reasons why.

PART 2

How you can fix things

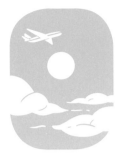

Shift work, time zones, jet lag

In an ideal world, we would go to sleep and wake in the morning with synchronised regularity, eating regularly, getting lots of daylight and exercise and relaxing before going to bed ... but life is life and we learn to adapt. However, it's worth considering the effects of unregulated day–night patterns and how best to minimise their effect.

Shift work

Disrupted sleep patterns affects around 18 per cent of all employees aged 15–64 in the EU who currently work shifts. While shift work suits many, there is an impact on health for most. Constantly trying to function outside the normal rhythms of your body clock has been linked to an increased risk of heart attack and stroke, obesity and type 2 diabetes. The chances of developing breast cancer rises from the European average of 1:9–2:9 among long-term shift workers.

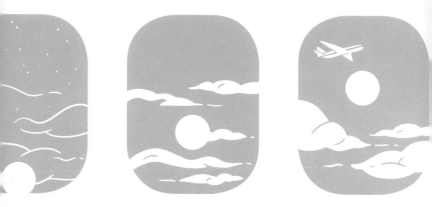

It doesn't sound a great lifestyle choice, does it? But if shift work is inevitable, then it's important to try and counterbalance it with enough sleep when possible, healthy eating, plus lots of daylight and exercise on days off.

Jet lag

Travelling across time zones – and back again quickly – can play havoc with our body clocks, leading to that well-known phenomenon, jet lag.

Jet lag is worse when you move from west to east because the body finds it harder to adapt to a shorter day than a longer one.

Tips to help reduce effects of jet lag

> Try and get as much normal sleep as possible before you travel so you are not exhausted before you arrive.
> Once aboard your flight, change your watch and phone to the time at your destination and start to work towards that in terms of eating and sleep.
> Keep hydrated – drink lots of water or coconut water, which contains five essential electrolytes: calcium, magnesium, potassium, sodium and phosphorus.
> Exposure to natural daylight helps the body adjust – staying awake during the day and going to bed when it's dark will help, even if it's out of sync, initially, with your body clock.

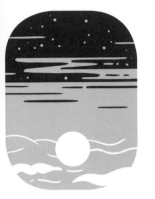 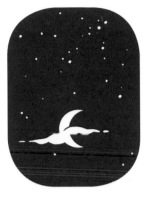 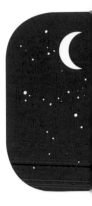

> Eat the following foods in the run up to your trip:
  - Cherries are a rich source of natural melatonin which can help regulate
  a new sleep pattern.
  - Brazil nuts, broccoli and other green vegetables, brown rice, fish and
  dairy products. These foods contain magnesium, which has a natural
  calming effect.
  - Avocados, turkey, cheese and milk as they contain tryptophan – another
  helpful sedative to aid sleep.

Social jet lag

The effects of social jet lag – disturbed sleep patterns, weakness and
disorientation – is pretty similar to the experience of actual jet lag. One
group who tend to experience this is teenagers (see page 51), partly because
there is often a discrepancy between the amount of sleep they need and the
amount they actually get.

For others – and this can happen to anyone, even those living a regular
life – it is the difference between the time your internal body clock thinks
it is and the time the outside world says it is. While society tells the time
from clocks, your body uses light and this can affect those of us who
have to adapt to the short days of winter and the longer days of summer.
Getting up early on a dark winter's morning, before your body is ready, can

leave you feeling tired and out of sorts.

Our 9–5, Monday to Friday working pattern, combined with late nights and lie-ins at weekends, is often behind this. Come Monday morning again, we have what researchers call 'social jet lag' where, for some, the difference can be the equivalent of taking a transatlantic flight on a Friday night and flying back on a Monday morning.

> **This [social jet lag] can confuse your body clock. The sense of tiredness than ensues is called post-sleep inertia, which can hang around for a few hours afterwards.**
> *Professor Jim Horne*

Polyphasic sleep

Rather than sleep in one block of sleep, once a day – the term for which is monophasic sleep – polyphasic sleep is a pattern of sleeping in numerous blocks throughout a 24-hour period, much as babies and infants do. This seems to have been more prevalent in historical times, before the invention of electric light when we were more dependent on natural daylight to live by.

In contrast to shift work, where sleep/wake cycles are constantly changing, one alleged benefit of regular polyphasic sleep/wake cycles is that this constantly refreshes the brain, allegedly making it more productive. It is possible to train ourselves to sleep in this way, as sailors at sea covering the night watch do. The United States military, said to spend millions of dollars on sleep research, train recruits in polyphasic sleep to ensure they can function fully day or night.

Leonardo da Vinci was said to sleep for only an hour and a half every day, taking 15-minute sleep breaks every four hours. He was phenomenally productive, achieving a huge artistic output of significant range and brilliance – but he is probably the exception that proves the rule and polyphasic sleep is counter-productive for most of us, causing the same symptoms of sleep deprivation that we experience from a general lack of sleep.

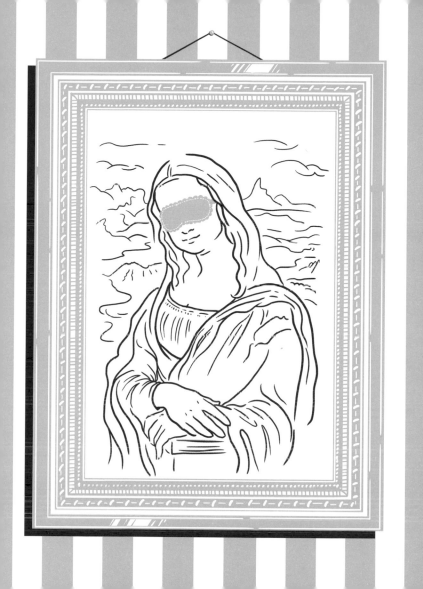

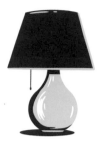

Insomnia

What is insomnia?

Most people think of insomnia as a straightforward inability to sleep. Technically, it is an inability to sleep well for at least three nights a week, for more than four weeks. The occasional bad night or two doesn't count as insomnia, more a blip in what is normal for you and is probably caused by external circumstances – jet lag, exam worry, temporary illness, for example – that are resolved fairly quickly.

> **A little insomnia is not without its value in making us appreciate sleep, in throwing a ray of light upon that darkness.** *Marcel Proust*

Symptoms of insomnia
> Inability to fall asleep – you feel tired, you go to bed, but your mind and body are still racing and, two hours later, you're exhausted but still awake.
> Constant waking – although you fall asleep reasonably easily, you wake several times a night and find it difficult to get back to sleep when you do.
> You fall asleep easily enough, sleep pretty well, but then wake early after a short night's sleep and can't sleep again – sometimes known as 'early morning waking'.
> Overall poor sleep quality – almost a combination of the first three descriptions.

For these symptoms to be classed as insomnia, rather than a one-off problem, they need to form a pattern over a period of weeks.

When is it a problem?
Whether or not insomnia is a problem for you will depend on a number of factors, but it mainly depends on how you feel and how well you are able to function with the sleep you get. We are all individual and while one person may cope quite well on six hours a night – possibly because they sleep very well when they do sleep – for others, it's too little and they need more.

For those who suffer from insomnia, and for whom the sleep they get is inadequate, it can cause feelings of irritability, lack of concentration, clumsiness through to causing accidents and health problems. Managing sleep and getting better sleep, which often means allowing more time to sleep, can contribute massively to overall health and well-being.

Paradoxically, insomnia can be related to sleep deprivation: the more tired we are, the more stress hormones kick in, and the more difficult it can be to relax and sleep well.

The good news is that there is much that can be done in terms of self-help before resorting to prescription medication – which can sometimes be helpful in the short term to break the pattern of insomnia.

The best cure for insomnia is to get a lot of sleep.

W.C. FIELDS

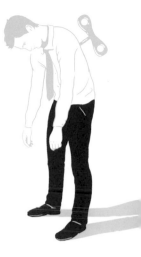

TATT & EDS

Tired All The Time and Excessive Daytime Sleepiness

Feeling tired all the time is a complaint often heard in a GP's surgery, so much so that it is a recognised syndrome, but teasing out its cause can be tricky and a first question will probably be about the amount and quality of sleep a patient is getting. However, in three-quarters of cases, a period of TATT is an isolated incident and any investigations seldom show an abnormal result.

Only when TATT is associated with other symptoms – significant weight loss, swollen lymph nodes, heart/lung disease, iron-deficiency anaemia or sleep apnoea – can a doctor do very much about insomnia as a symptom.

Anaemia

Feelings of fatigue and tiredness can be caused by a lack of iron in the diet: iron-deficiency anaemia. Heavy periods in women or a diet poor in iron-rich foods (meat, spinach, watercress, kale, eggs, dried apricots etc), can be

Symptoms of sleep apnoea

› Excessive daytime sleepiness.
› Morning headaches.
› Recent weight gain.
› Awakening in the morning not feeling rested.
› Waking at night feeling confused.
› Change in your level of attention, concentration, or memory.
› Observed pauses in breathing during sleep.

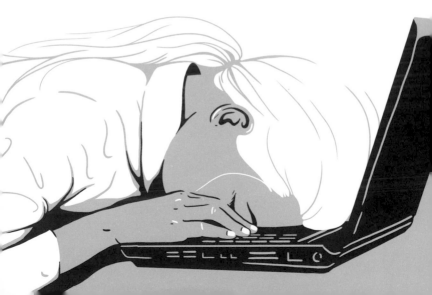

a cause, but it is easily rectified. Certainly, if you suspect this to be a cause of tiredness, it's worth a quick blood test to check for haemoglobin levels in the blood, improve the diet or take an iron supplement for a while. Be sure to include additional vitamin C in your diet to help with iron absorption, too.

Sleep apnoea

Sleep apnoea, sometimes known as obstructive sleep disorder, is often associated with being overweight and snoring loudly at night. Apnoea means to stop breathing, which is effectively what happens briefly when the breathing is blocked, and when this happens, a lack of oxygen causes a shift from deep sleep to light sleep or wakefulness, in order to restore normal breathing. These constant interruptions throughout the night can occur several times an hour.

EDS

Excessive Daytime Sleepiness (EDS) or hypersomnia can also occur for a variety of reasons – sleep apnoea and restless legs syndrome among them. However, it can also occur among those who appear to be sleeping well and for long enough, for no known reason – this is described as being idiopathic – and can be more difficult to fix. This is comparatively uncommon and not usually caused by disordered sleeping. As well as taking naps during the day, most people with the disorder sleep for more than 10 hours a night and struggle to wake in the morning because they feel very drowsy and confused, even though the quality of their sleep is generally fine.

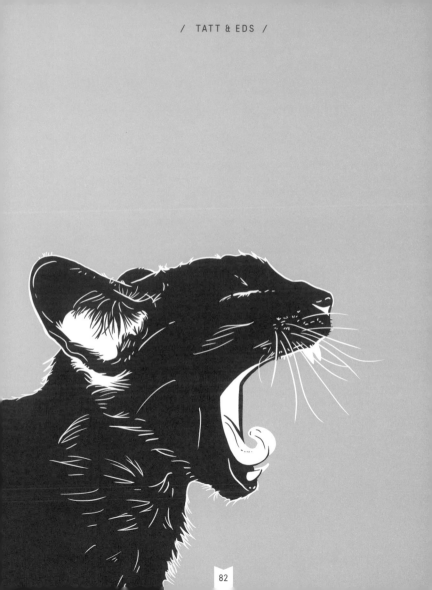

Yawning

We think we yawn because we are tired or bored. But scientists have
come to some interesting conclusions about the phenomenon of the yawn.
It turns out that it isn't directly related to how much sleep we've had or
how physically tired we are – although, paradoxically, we do tend to yawn
when we feel subjectively sleepy and it does increase when bored – but
we also do it when we're hungry. It is often seen as a sign of lethargy and
ennui and interpreted as such – remember Sasha Obama's infamous yawn
during her father's 2013 inaugural address? – but this apparent cause and
effect is subtly different in reality.

Yawning is, in fact, rooted in the primal centre of the brain that falls
outside our conscious control and, as neuroscientist Robert Provine
suggests, we do it automatically in an effort to re-engage our bodies
and minds, to transition from one behavioural state to another: sleep to
wakefulness, wakefulness to sleep, anxiety to calm, boredom to alertness.

As part of Provine's research, he looked at the incidence of yawning
among soldiers about to parachute from a plane: the incidence of yawning
went markedly up as they moved towards to the door just prior to their
jump. In an effort to gather focus and the alertness required, they yawned.
And this yawning was the subtle, but often misinterpreted, trigger toward
full engagement. A shaking up and refocus. A survival mechanism.

And why is yawning contagious? Why do we yawn when we see another
person yawn? Apparently we do it out of empathy, a sort of social bonding,
in subconscious recognition that we may need a bit of a prod, or food, or
something to keep us going. All at a deeply primal level, of course.

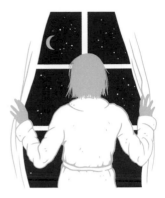

What's stopping you sleeping?

You may have always been a light sleeper, prone to occasional insomnia. Or you may have been a good sleeper all your life, suddenly hit by bouts of wakefulness and fitful sleep. Whatever your situation or sleep history, it's sometimes worth running through a checklist of what might be disturbing you or stopping you from sleeping and reviewing what could be causing your sleep patterns to be changing.

> **We are such stuff as dreams are made on; and our little life is rounded with a sleep.** *William Shakespeare*

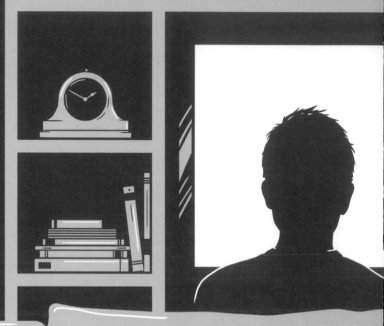

Light

During the day, lots of exposure to full-spectrum light (essentially daylight, but in winter months using a lamp with full-spectrum light bulb will help), helps set your body clock. This needs to be counteracted at night by reducing exposure to light as you head towards sleep.

Although any type of light stops you feeling sleepy, research has shown that light towards the blue end of the spectrum is especially effective at keeping you awake because – as we know – it suppresses the production of melatonin. Unfortunately, computer screens, tablets, smartphones, flat-screen televisions and LED lighting all

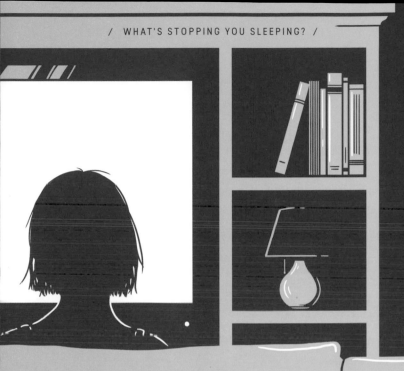

emit large amounts of blue light, and so it's important to avoid them before bedtime. According to research carried out by Professor Richard Wiseman, around 80 per cent of people routinely use these devices running up to bedtime, and among 18- to 24-year-olds this figure increases to a remarkable 91 per cent.

Amber-tinted glasses can cut out glare, and it's also possible to fit screens with commercially produced blue-light-blocking filters. Another solution, of course, is to avoid all electronic devices that can be over-stimulating in other ways, and take deliberate steps to introduce sleep-inducing strategies into bedtime routines.

Alcohol

That alcohol interferes with the normal sleep process is a well-established fact. Drinking a lot of alcohol just prior to going to bed means that sleep patterns are disrupted: you fall immediately into deep sleep, missing out on the usual first, REM stage of sleep (see page 23).

'Deep sleep is when the body restores itself, and alcohol can interfere with this,' says Dr John Shneerson, head of Papworth Hospital's Sleep Centre in the UK. 'As the alcohol starts to wear off, your body can come out of deep sleep and back into REM sleep, which is much easier to wake from. That's why you often wake up after just a few hours sleep when you've been drinking.'

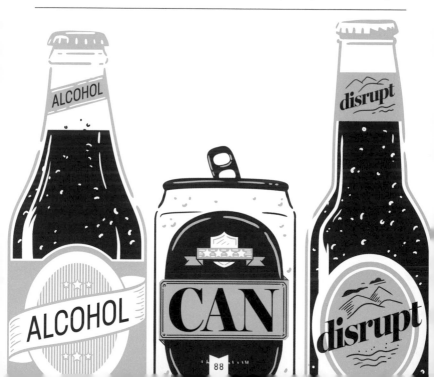

Six to seven cycles of REM sleep is what should be normal during the night, leaving you feeling refreshed when you wake. However, if you've been drinking alcohol, it's more typical to only experience one or two cycles of REM sleep – which may result in you feeling exhausted when you wake.

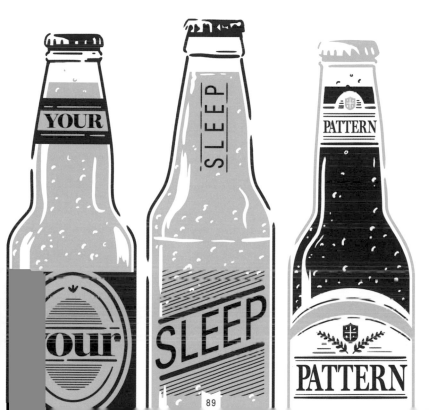

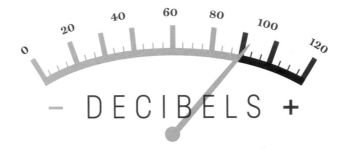

Laugh and the world laughs with you, snore and you sleep alone.

ANTHONY BURGESS

Snoring

Snoring is increasingly being recognised as a health problem, not only because the noise of it might keep your sleeping partner awake, but also because it can contribute to daytime sleepiness or other problems.

How? Well, snoring occurs when the muscles of the throat relax, close in slightly and vibrate as we breathe – the noise of the snore is an attempt to get air in and out of the lungs. Sleeping on your back, being overweight, drinking alcohol, allergies, enlarged tonsils or nasal polyps can all contribute to problems with snoring, and eliminating these physical problems can often alleviate snoring.

While mild or intermittent snoring is no problem – even though it can be an irritant to a sleeping partner – it is when snoring becomes a symptom of airway obstruction that disturbs us (even if we don't notice it), by constantly breaking and disrupting the normal sleep cycle – it can be a symptom of sleep apnoea. This, in turn, can lead to TATT and EDS (see page 79) and needs addressing.

Hunger

It may seem a little ridiculous to cite hunger as a cause of sleep problems in our over-fed world, but if you eat a light, early supper at around 6 p.m. without anything else before bed, you may find yourself waking at 5 a.m. with a rumbling stomach. It's not so much your stomach rumbling that will wake you, but the kicking-in of the hormone cortisol, needed to release stored carbohydrates in your body, as your blood sugar level falls. Cortisol is also a stress hormone, and it might be this that wakes you as it gears your body up toward activity. If you suffer early morning waking, you may want to have a light, sleep-inducing snack – a milky drink, oat cake and peanut butter, or a banana or other slow-release carbohydrate snack – before you go to bed, to allow your body to sleep well.

Pain

Physical discomfort and pain, either in the long or short term, can disrupt sleep. Taking painkillers before bed may be one solution, but this needs to be weighed up against other pain-reducing measures. It's also worth checking the quality of the mattress, which may be too hard or too soft, and whether the pillow is giving adequate neck support. Back pain can be eased by sleeping with a pillow between the knees, which also takes the pressure off knee joints.

Restless Legs Syndrome (RLS) is worth a mention here because, if not exactly painful, it can cause sleep disorders and insomnia, purely because it creates unpleasant sensations in the legs and a strong urge to move them – which is worse at night.

Stress, Anxiety, Depression

It's sometimes difficult to know which came first, the psychological or the sleep problem, as the two can be closely linked.

Lack of sleep can make you feel out of sorts, anxious, stressed or depressed in the short term, and when it becomes a chronic problem, it can be difficult to find a solution.

Having said that, it's worth tackling the two together: improve your sleep and your psychological problems become more manageable, while improving your levels of stress can help relieve the anxiety and depression that are hindering sleep.

IT'S ALWAYS WORTH TAKING IMMEDIATE STEPS TO ADDRESS ANY MENTAL HEALTH CONCERNS

› Breathing and visualisation exercises help refocus away from sources of stress: practice relaxation breathing techniques (see page 101) while visualising a peaceful, happy time.

› Exercise is good for both physical and mental health as it provides an outlet for frustrations while releasing mood-enhancing endorphins. Balance more active exercise with something like yoga or swimming, which can be particularly effective at reducing anxiety and stress.

› Make a to-do list, but prioritise realistically, spending your time and energy on those things that are truly important. Break up large projects into smaller, more easily managed, tasks and delegate where you can.

› Use soft, calming music to relax your mind and body, and lower your blood pressure.

› Don't skimp on sleep – it recharges your brain and improves focus, concentration and mood, all of which makes life easier to manage.

› Try not to let thoughts go round and round in your head: volunteer in your community or offer help to a friend or neighbour. Helping others helps to take our minds off our own anxiety.

› Don't try to cope alone if things feel overwhelming: talk to someone and consider seeing a doctor or therapist for help.

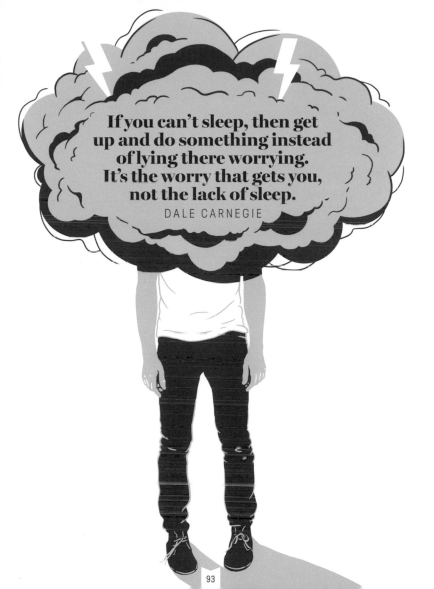

If you can't sleep, then get up and do something instead of lying there worrying. It's the worry that gets you, not the lack of sleep.

DALE CARNEGIE

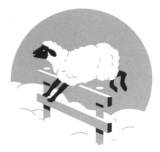

Sleep solutions

Having established what might be hindering you from getting good or adequate sleep, and having taken practical steps to fix things, what other sleep solutions might help?

Counting sheep

Let's get this one out of the way. The principle on which this old recommendation is based is a simple relaxation and mind-clearing trick. focusing on visualising sheep and counting them, one by one, is the sort of mindless activity that can take your mind off other mind-stimulating thoughts. For some it works, while for others it's not enough to do the trick of stopping other thoughts from popping up. If that's you, try counting backwards from one thousand in sevens: i.e. 1,000, 993, 986, 979, etc., instead.

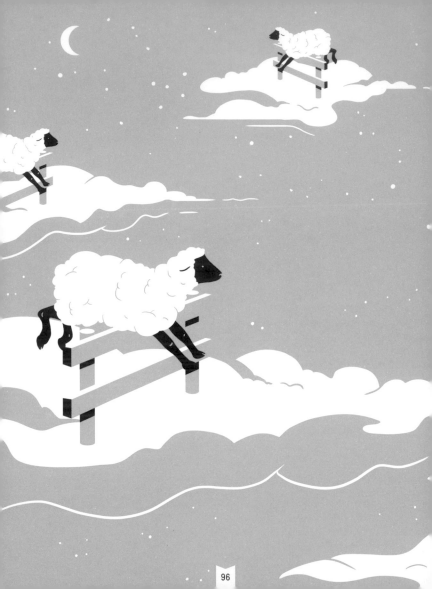

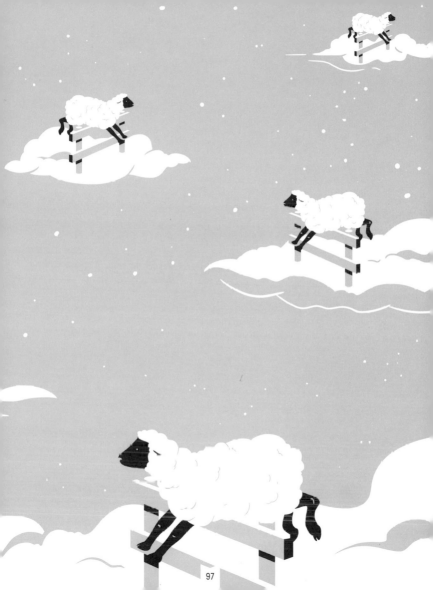

Natural sedatives

> *Chamomile:* Two types of chamomile are used for health purposes, renowned for their soothing and sleep-inducing effect – German chamomile (*Matricaria retutica*) and Roman, or English, chamomile (*Chamaemelum nobile*). The dried flower heads can be infused in water to make a tisane or tea, and commercial tea bags are readily available in supermarkets.

> *Valerian:* Another herb, valerian (*Valeriana officinalis*), is also available as an over the counter herbal remedy from the chemist, and has long been used as an antidote to stress and anxiety and as a sleep aid. It seems to increase the function of GABA (gamma-aminobutyric acid) in the brain, which is a neurotransmitter that has a calming effect on the nervous system and muscles. Without it, we remain tense and over-stimulated and often find it difficult to 'switch off'.

> *Lavender:* Of all the herbs renowned for its calming effect, lavender (*Lavandula angustifolia*) is probably the most well known. Its lovely scent, redolent of sunny summer afternoons, comes from the flowers and the leaves, with lavender oil extracted from the flowers, or dried to use in an infusion of tea. The dried flowers can be used in lavender bags and the oil can be added to massage oil or a warm bath.

> *Tryptophan:* Tryptophan is an essential amino acid that can be found in various foods. Tryptophan combines with vitamin B_6, transforming into serotonin and niacin in the liver and, once in circulation, the pineal gland uses it to make melatonin – that sleep-inducing hormone we know and love. Foods high in tryptophan include poultry, milk products, cereal grains, avocados, pumpkin (squash) and chickpeas (garbanzos).

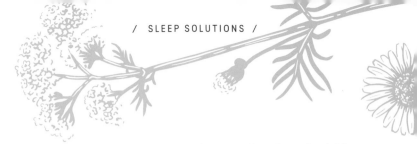

> **Magnesium:** Magnesium is a mineral we are often short of and this can have a direct impact on our ability to relax and sleep as it is essential for the function of GABA (see opposite). Whether the brain is in off or on mode is affected by neurochemicals like noradrenaline, serotonin and histamine, and these need to be kept in check by GABA: too much of the former without the latter and we are too hyped up to sleep.

Excessive adrenaline and stress, often in abundance in the sleep deprived, are believed to drain magnesium from the body. Magnesium is also necessary for the body to bind adequate amounts of serotonin, a mood-elevating chemical within the brain that creates a feeling of well-being and relaxation.

According to the *Journal of the American College of Nutrition*, 68 per cent of US adults consume less than the Recommended Daily Allowance (RDA) of magnesium, but what symptoms might you have if this is the cause of your wakefulness? If you're having difficulty in going to sleep or find that you wake early in spite of sleeping badly, you may be deficient. Regular muscular cramps can be an indication, along with having cold hands and feet and experiencing tight muscles in the neck and shoulders. You may even notice muscle twitches, in the eyelid, for example.

Good food sources for magnesium include green leafy vegetables, wheatgerm, pumpkin seeds and almonds. A supplement of 400–500 mg at night can help, but check with your doctor first as it can interact with many different medications, and too much of it can have an adverse effect. If you take a supplement, opt for magnesium citrate or ascorbate rather than magnesium oxide, which can cause diarrhoea in sensitive people. For some, transdermal magnesium (outlined below) is the best way to take it, especially as we age and our digestive absorption is less good.

> **Epsom salts:** Epsom salts are a form of magnesium that can be added to a warm bath before bed. Studies have shown that transdermal

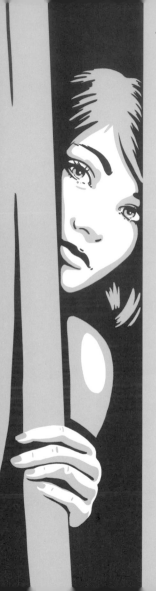

absorption increases levels in the body, helping to relax muscular tension too.

› ***5-HTP:*** 5-Hydroxytryptophan (5-HTP) is sometimes recommended for sleep, or added to natural sleep aids, because it is a natural amino acid that is a precursor to both tryptophan, which we know helps sleep, and also serotonin, which is a natural mood enhancer, produced by the brain and the gut. However there's not a great deal of clinical evidence to say it will work, but it might be worth a try and is sometimes included in natural health preparations alongside vitamin B6 and melatonin.

› ***Ear plugs:*** If you are easily disturbed by external noise at night – your partner's snores or the dawn chorus as the day breaks – use ear plugs. Soft wax or silicone ones that can be moulded to comfortably fit and exclude noise work much better than the hard foam ones given out on long-haul flights.

› ***Black-out curtains:*** Making your bedroom adequately dark is essential if you have trouble sleeping as light stops the production of the sleep hormone melatonin. Curtains or blinds that really cut out light make a huge difference, especially if the early morning light of a summer's dawn also wakes you.

› ***Herb pillow:*** Make your own herb pillow as a sleep aid. It needn't be large, 30 x 15 cm (12 x 6 in) is fine. Use soft, loosely woven cotton fabric for the inner pocket and stuff it with dried chamomile flower heads, lavender and hops before sewing together. Make an outer cover from more finely woven cotton, or silk, with ties at the outer end, and sleep with it on your pillow.

RELAXATION BREATHING EXERCISE

> Find a comfortable position, perhaps lying on your back with a small pillow to support your head, your knees bent and arms and hands relaxed. Tuck your neck in, lengthening the back of your neck – what Alexander Technique teachers call the constructive rest position.

> Consciously relax your shoulders by scrunching them up to your ears and then dropping them down again, feeling heavy and relaxed against the floor or bed on which you're lying. Consciously relax other muscles that might be feeling tense.

> Ensure you're warm enough and comfortable.

> Close your eyes.

> Gently breathe in through your nose, concentrating on keeping the flow even without forcing it at all. Pause for a moment before breathing out through your mouth.

> This may feel odd at first, even a little strained, but stay with it until it feels more harmonious.

> As you begin to breathe a little deeper, you will take in more oxygen and this will slow your breathing, even making the pauses between breaths a little longer. This is normal. The trigger for our breathing is the level of carbon dioxide in the blood, which will fall as we breathe more calmly and deeply and take in more oxygen. Let this process happen naturally.

> Continue breathing in this way, keeping your attention focused on the in breath, the pause and then the out breath, finding your own rhythm.

> If you find it difficult to focus just on the breathing, it sometimes helps to silently intone 'in' on the in breath, and 'out' on the out breath.

> Alternatively, to help you focus, visualise a small pebble dropping into a pool of water and sinking to the bottom with each breath.

It will take practice at first to become familiar with this calm way of breathing, but in time it can become a useful tool to lead you into relaxation, sleep or any meditative practice.

Make a list

Rather than constantly running through everything you want to remember the next day, but are afraid you might forget, make a list. Then you can stop worrying about forgetting something, relax and sleep.

The main facts in human life are five: birth, food, sleep, love and death. *E. M. Forster*

Music

Music can aid sleep in a number of ways. One is as low, background 'white' noise that blocks out other noise; another is as part of a winding-down routine that leads to sleep, much as parents sing lullabies to their children. But it can also be used to encourage those brain waves that are a precursor to sleep.

If you've ever had a spa treatment to the accompaniment of plinkety-plonk, wind chimes and wave music, or the metallic ring of Tibetan singing bowls, designed to lull you toward relaxation – this is music that links to your own brain waves.

We move between Alpha (between 7 and 12 Hz) and Beta (13 and 40 Hz) waves when awake – and very occasionally Gamma (above 40 Hz), but only when actively problem solving or under acute stress – and the Delta (0 and 4 Hz) waves of deep sleep via the more elusive Theta (4 and 7 Hz) brain waves as we drift off.

In order to access specific brain waves, it's possible to include binaural beats into music that correlate to specific brain waves. That's why dance music that includes Beta binaural beats can make you feel upbeat and energised and, conversely, Alpha and Delta binaural beats are found in music specifically marketed as an aid to meditation, relaxation or sleep.

Cognitive Behaviour Therapy (CBT)

CBT is increasingly recognised as being helpful for insomnia and other sleep-related problems that have been ongoing for more than four weeks. CBT involves looking at how thought processes (cognition) affect

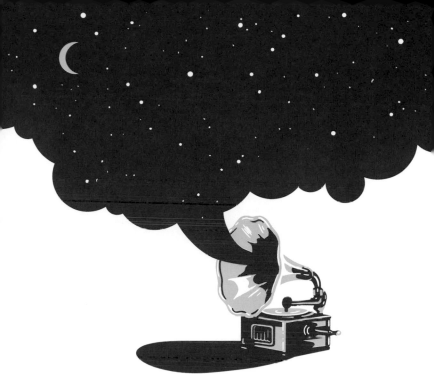

And the night shall be filled with music, and the cares that infest the day shall fold their tents like the Arabs and as silently steal away.

HENRY WADSWORTH LONGFELLOW

behaviour and how, by changing the thoughts we have, we can alter and improve what we do or how we experience life.

In terms of how this might help with insomnia, it's a way of looking at some of the thought processes that occur, i.e., 'I can't sleep, I'll never sleep, I won't be able to cope tomorrow without sleep.', that can actually inhibit the behaviours that encourage sleep. If you lie awake in bed, staring at the clock, tensely thinking, 'I can't sleep', then it can become a self-fulfilling prophecy.

Learning how to resist panicky thoughts and substitute them with a revised belief that sleep will be possible, that you will get enough sleep and all will be well, can take time but has been proven to work well in combination with other sleep hygiene (see page 117).

A key part of CBT when used for this purpose is to understand the process of sleep and to revisit some of the myths and misconceptions that surround it. Sleep hygiene is another important component and you may be asked to keep a sleep diary (see page 113). Following four or five sessions with a specially trained health professional, most people are able to restore

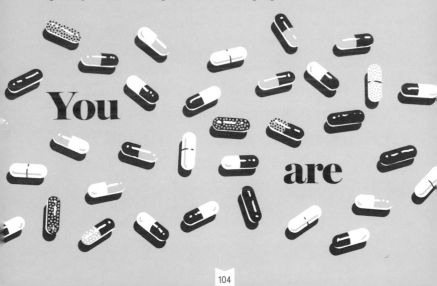

You are

good sleep and learn a new and effective way of managing occasional and intermittent insomnia in the future.

Sleep medication

Apart from over-the-counter remedies like valerian or antihistamines, your doctor may sometimes prescribe a short course of sleeping tablets in order to alleviate the immediate symptom of insomnia while also addressing any other factors that may be contributing to a sleeping problem.

In the nineteenth century, opium was a popular cure for sleeplessness – the British didn't go to war with the Chinese for nothing – and laudanum, a tincture of alcohol and morphine, was easily and readily available to those who could afford it. Cannabis was also used, although this was considered more dangerous than laudanum, and Queen Victoria's personal physician, Dr J. R. Reynolds, prescribed it for her to 'assist sleep during menstrual cramps'. In an article in *The Lancet*, 1890, he also reflected that it was 'one of the most valuable medicines we possess for treating insomnia'.

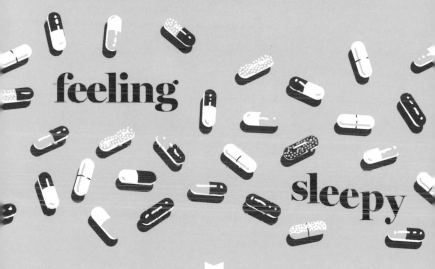

feeling sleepy

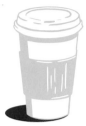

Crisis Management Plan

If you have hit crisis point with poor sleep or insomnia, or if you want to take the first steps towards improving sleep, this is for you. Remember that what you do during the day will have an impact on your night-time sleep, so this *plan* takes into account the 24-hour day.

Alarm clock

However badly you slept, set your alarm for a morning start and force yourself out of bed. Your wake-up call is your first body clock clue for regulating sleep.

You can also set an alarm for the evening – to remind you that it is time to get ready to go to bed.

Breakfast

Eat a light, nutritious breakfast that includes protein. Egg on toast is good; muesli with oats, nuts and fruit is too. Again, eating breakfast helps regulate your body clock and, if you balance protein with carbohydrates, you'll avoid blood sugar hikes and dips that can contribute to feeling tired.

Caffeine

Caffeine – whether from coffee, Coke or tea is fine – up until 3 p.m. After this point, ban it from your lips. In any event, limit your intake to one or two cups daily; or avoid it altogether if sleep has become completely elusive. Bear in mind that it can take your body time to adjust: going from six cups a day to nil might cause withdrawal symptoms initially. Cut down slowly over the course of a week to minimise the effects of this.

Caffeine content

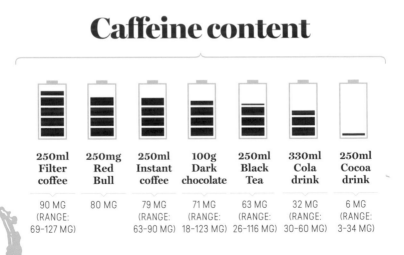

250ml Filter coffee	250mg Red Bull	250ml Instant coffee	100g Dark chocolate	250ml Black Tea	330ml Cola drink	250ml Cocoa drink
90 MG (RANGE: 69-127 MG)	80 MG	79 MG (RANGE: 63-90 MG)	71 MG (RANGE: 18-123 MG)	63 MG (RANGE: 26-116 MG)	32 MG (RANGE: 30-60 MG)	6 MG (RANGE: 3-34 MG)

(SOURCE: INTERNATIONAL FOOD INFORMATION COUNCIL)

Napping

If, after your early start, you need to recharge your batteries mid-afternoon, then take no more than a 20-minute nap. You should ensure it's no longer and take it before 4 p.m., to avoid reducing your ability to fall asleep later.

Exercise

This will also help both tire and relax you physically. Even if it's only a brisk 20-minute walk to and from work, it will pay dividends. However, if you are in the habit of taking more strenuous exercise, at the gym, on the tennis court, football pitch or taking a run, the optimum time for your body, your body clock and to support sleep, is between 3 p.m. and 6 p.m.

What and when to eat before sleep

Eating too early can cause early morning waking as blood sugar levels fall, triggering cortisol release, which can wake you. Eating too heavily, too late in the evening can also be counter-productive. Ideally you don't want to leave more than 10–12 hours between your last meal – or snack – and waking up.

Choose sleep-inducing foods, foods high in tryptophan – poultry, milk products, cereal grains, avocados, pumpkin (squash), chickpeas (garbanzos), walnuts. Also include foods containing magnesium and vitamin B in your evening meal. If you have eaten earlier and need a snack, try a banana and a milky drink.

Alcohol

Avoid alcohol altogether if you have hit crisis point, as this can cause waking and fractured sleep as it disturbs your normal sleep phases and may make you wake in the night with a full bladder. Although a depressant, alcohol demands too much of the body and conflicts with peaceful sleep.

Sleep environment

Make sure the room in which you sleep is quiet, dark and neither too hot nor too cold. Fit black-out blinds or curtains, use ear plugs if necessary (soft, malleable wax or silicone ones are best).

Electronic equipment

Prohibit the use of anything that emits blue light – computer, smartphone, laptop and iPad screens – for up to two hours before trying to sleep, because it prevents the normal secretion of sleep-inducing melatonin.

Pain

Acute or chronic physical pain can prevent you falling asleep if you're not comfortable in bed, or cause waking. Take steps to reduce pain; consult your doctor or physiotherapist, or use an over-the-counter painkiller in the short term.

Warm feet

Cold feet can keep you awake, but bed socks solve this problem for many or, alternatively, have a warm bath before bed.

Stop

Stop all work three hours before bed. Eat, wind down and relax. Use a bedtime routine to prepare for bed, but only go to bed when you feel sleepy. Read a book or listen to relaxing music, making sure that your bedside light isn't too bright.

Relax

Spend time with a cup of chamomile tea in a bath scented with lavender having eaten a banana – sounds crazy, but works for some – and then sleep on a pillow stuffed with hops and lavender. Use breathing techniques (see page 101) to help you prepare for sleep.

I want to sleep by Harriet Griffey

First published in 2015 by Hardie Grant Books

Hardie Grant Books (UK)
5th & 6th Floors
52–54 Southwark Street
London SE1 1UN
www.hardiegrant.co.uk

Hardie Grant Books (Australia)
Ground Floor, Building 1
658 Church Street
Melbourne, VIC 3121
www.hardiegrant.com.au

The moral rights of Harriet Griffey to be identified as the author
of this work have been asserted by her in accordance with the
Copyright, Designs and Patents Act 1988.

Text © Harriet Griffey

All rights reserved. No part of this publication may be reproduced,
stored in a retrieval system or transmitted in any form by any
means, electronic, electrostatic, magnetic tape, mechanical,
photocopying, recording or otherwise, without
the prior written permission of the Publisher.

British Library Cataloguing-in-Publication Data. A catalogue record
for this book is available from the British Library.

ISBN: 978-174270-931-4

Publisher: Kate Pollard
Senior Editor: Kajal Mistry
Editors: Nicky Jeanes and Louise Francis
Cover and Internal Design: Julia Murray
Colour Reproduction by p2d

Printed and bound in China by 1010

10 9 8 7 6 5 4

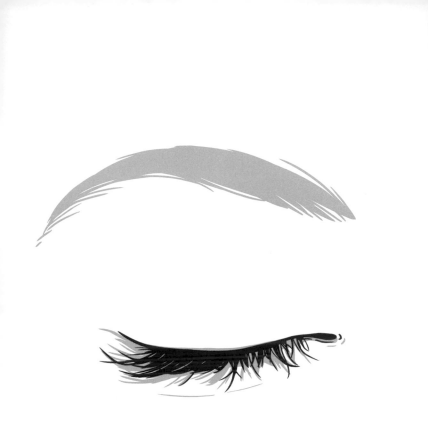

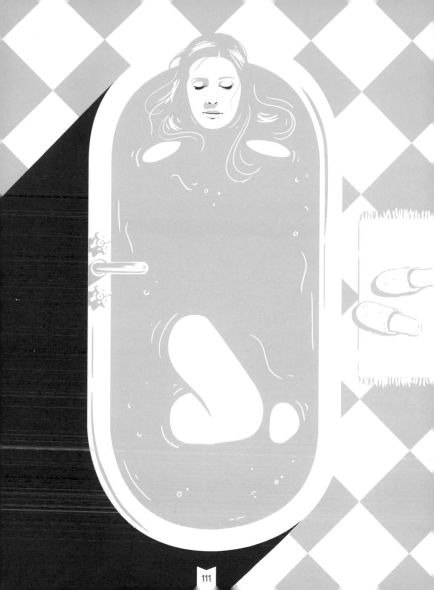

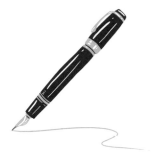

Assessing the problem: keeping a sleep diary

When you are trying to identify the causes of your tiredness, insomnia or poor sleep, it's sometimes worth keeping a sleep diary for a period of time. Only in retrospect can some contributory patterns of behaviour be identified. It will also give you some concrete information with which you can approach your doctor for help, if you are unable to improve things yourself and need help.

_____

_____

_____

_____

Every day, make a record of the following:
> **Awake time:** whether woken naturally, using an alarm clock or woken by some external event.
> **How you felt**
> **Main, non-routine event of the day:** i.e. work presentation, social event, or other.
> **Meals:** times of breakfast, lunch, last meal of the day, etc.
> **What you did before going to bed**
> **Time you went to bed**
> **Time you went to sleep**
> **Total amount of sleep:** including periods of sleep within that – i.e. six hours, woke twice.
> **Any other information:** i.e. illness or accident, exceptional event, etc.

It's important to consider your sleep as part of your 24-hour day, so keep a sleep diary for a couple of weeks, long enough to see if any patterns emerge and also to establish whether you have a true insomnia or whether it's what you're doing that is causing your sleep problem.

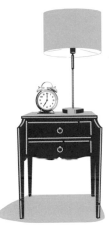

Sleep hygiene

'Sleep hygiene' is the term used by health professionals to describe the general practice that helps to promote good sleep habits. The three main aspects of sleep hygiene to be considered, when making changes to improve or re-establish good sleep patterns, are the environment in which you sleep, exercise and diet. Again, this relates to the 24-hour day – what you do during your waking hours will have an effect on how you sleep.

Sleeping environment

The bedroom should be a place of sleep, not work or entertainment. While some can tolerate a combination of uses for their bedroom, if you have trouble sleeping it is worth keeping the bedroom associated purely with sleep rather than watching television, playing video games, doing emails on a laptop or texting friends. Not only are these activities too stimulating for some before sleep, the blue light from electronic gadgets will inhibit the production of sleep-inducing melatonin.

Your bed should be a place of comfort, not too hard or soft, hot or cold, or crowded. If you find your partner disruptive, consider a larger bed or even separate beds for sleeping. There is nothing worse for a light sleeper to be constantly disturbed by someone else's shufflings or mutterings, temperature clashes or tussles over the duvet.

Ideally, the temperature in a bedroom should be around 65°F (18°C) and unstuffy. If you can't have a window open, leave the door ajar to allow air to circulate.

An ioniser in the bedroom may help sleep. Air particles are electrically neutral but become positive from dust, pollution, pollen, synthetic fibres and central heating and this can cause problems with tension, irritability and daytime headaches in sensitive people. Charging the air with negative ions helps counteract this.

Keep bedside lights low, enough to read by but no brighter, and if you must use a Kindle to read, turn the light to low, too.

Charles Dickens always insisted on sleeping with his head pointing north and to ensure he did so, never travelled anywhere without a compass. According to some ancient esoteric principles, sleeping in this position guards against insomnia and this is, apparently, why Dickens went to such lengths to ensure his sleeping position, although the notion of insomnia didn't exist until later.

Exercise

Why will exercising help you sleep? It helps tire you physically, which, given so many of us have very sedentary lives, isn't so easy to do. It eases muscular tension and counteracts the effect of stress hormones on our bodies and, by extension, our minds. It's a distraction: when we are focused on exercising our bodies, it stops repetitive and stressful thought patterns. It also releases mood-enhancing endorphins.

So regular daytime exercise will help you sleep – it doesn't have to be a hard gym workout, or a game of football, even a brisk 20-minute daily walk will help.

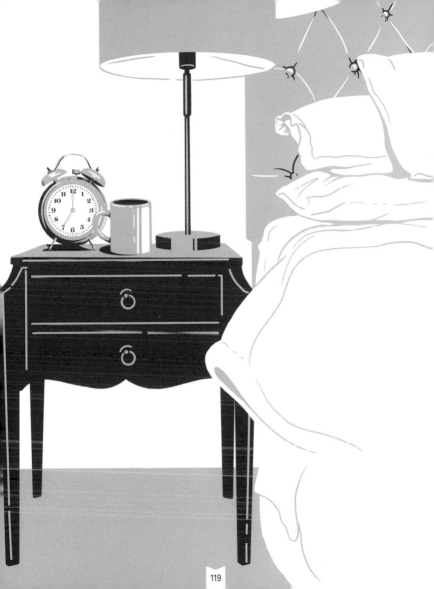

The only proviso is, when it comes to sleep, don't exercise too late in the day – not after 7 p.m., unless it's gentle exercise like yoga or swimming, as physical exertion raises the core temperature and over-stimulates you physically.

Eating and drinking

Regular meals not only keep your body stable, they also keep your body clock happy. The process of eating and digesting food is one of the cues that help us regulate our days and differentiate our day from night. Eating also takes energy, even while it provides it, and if you eat a large, nutritionally complex meal less than four hours before you want to sleep, it will probably keep you awake.

That said, if you eat a light supper six hours before bedtime it may not be enough to keep you asleep all night. In some, the dip in blood sugar after 6–8 hours can release cortisol, a stress hormone that may wake you early. A light snack or milky drink before bed may be enough to make the difference.

Bedtime routine

There is enormous value to having a bedtime routine for small children – it helps them wind down and prepare for sleep – but we forget that we also need to ensure a winding-down period and having a routine of sorts helps us, too.

If you are struggling with sleep and have no routine, incorporating one will help. Aim to follow the pointers of the Crisis Management Plan, especially those that focus on the end of the day (see page 107).

Don't expect any change you make to work immediately. It can take some time for your body to learn to relax and wind down and you won't necessarily sleep better straight away but, if you trust the process and allow it time, it will help you. Remember, it always takes time to break old habits and introduce new ones.

Create a routine

| Stop work at least three hours before bed. | Eat your last meal no later than four hours before bed. | Have a relaxing bath – add Epsom salts and lavender oil to the water. | Dim the lights. | Read a book or listen to relaxing music. |

Routines may include taking a warm bath or a relaxing walk in the evening, or practicing meditation/relaxation exercises. Psychologically, the completion of such a practice tells your mind and body that the day's work is over and you are free to relax and sleep.

ANDREW WEIL

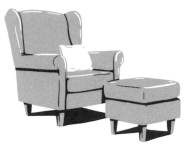

Napping

It's official – taking a nap can be good for you

Even if the language we use suggests that taking a nap is an illicit activity
– caught napping, stealing forty winks, snoozing – current thinking is that
it's actually good for you.

Take a rest. A field that is rested gives a beautiful crop. *Ovid*

It seems that our continental cousins know the value of the siesta. In 2009,
sleep researcher Kimberly Cote from Brock University in Canada reviewed
the vast amount of psychological work into napping and concluded that
even the shortest of naps made significant improvements in people's mood,
reaction times and general alertness.

Access those Alpha waves

The benefit of the nap isn't so much about making up for lost night-time sleep, it's more to do with refreshing neurological activity and re-accessing those brain waves that help cohesive thought. In an ideal world, we'd be utilising our Alpha brain waves to function, where we show a relaxed but effortless alertness, and focus and concentration are easy. However, in the course of a busy morning's work, we might shift gear to Beta waves, dealing with the stress of a difficult commute to work, deadlines and interruptions, and this has a negative effect on our ability to concentrate and focus. A nap shifts us into Theta waves for 20-minutes, which restores those calm, alert Alpha waves when we wake.

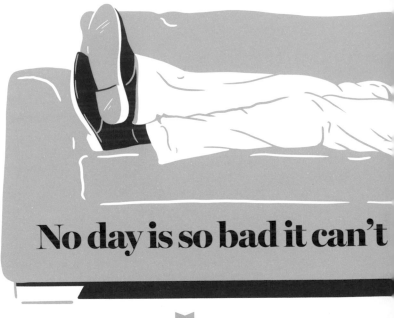

No day is so bad it can't

Research by NASA revealed that pilots who take a 20-minute nap in the cockpit (with a co-pilot taking over the controls!) are subsequently 35 per cent more alert and twice as focused as those that didn't nap.

Good for your heart

A recent six-year study into napping by Harvard University looked at the lives of more than 20,000 adults aged between 20 and 80. All participants were asked about their dietary habits, levels of physical exercise and – importantly – the extent to which they napped. Even after taking into account age and level of physical activity, those who took a 30-minute siesta at least three times a week had a 37 per cent lower risk of heart-related death.

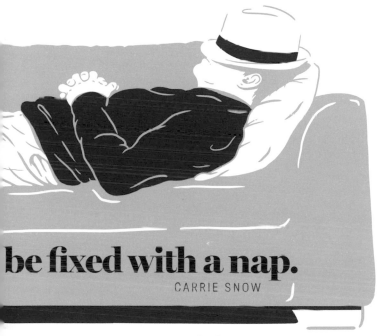

be fixed with a nap.
CARRIE SNOW

Good for your memory

Even the shortest of naps can have a surprisingly big impact on your memory, too. In 2008, scientists from the University of Dusseldorf asked volunteers to memorise a list of words and then randomly allocated them to one of three groups. The first group remained awake, the second slept for about 40 minutes and the third took a six-minute nap. When asked to recall the words, the first group did OK, the 40-minute sleepers did better, but those who had taken a six-minute nap did best of all.

You must sleep sometime between lunch and dinner, and no half-way measures. Take off your clothes and get into bed. That's what I always do. Don't think you will be doing less work because you sleep during the day. That's a foolish notion held by people who have no imaginations. You will be able to accomplish more. You get two days in one – well, at least one and a half.
Winston Churchill

Even if we don't quite follow Churchill's routine – his was devised during a time of national crisis, don't forget, when he spent long night-time hours in a wartime bunker under Whitehall – you should get rid of any lingering doubts about whether or not napping is a good use of time. It is also useful to know what time is best for you to take a nap and this correlates to the body's circadian rhythms that affect our energy levels through the day. So it's best to time your nap when you have a natural energy slump and that depends on what time you woke.

There is more refreshment and stimulation in a nap, even of the briefest, than in all the alcohol ever distilled. *Edward Lucas*

Don't worry if you don't fall asleep. Research shows that even just lying down with the intention of napping is enough to cause a healthy reduction in your blood pressure. And if you need to feel wide awake directly after having a short nap, drink a cup of coffee or other caffeinated drink just before dozing off. The caffeine will start to work its magic about 25 minutes later – just as you are waking up.

For optimum effect, however, naps should be just that – a nap – rather than a full, 90-minute cycle of sleep. Power naps of 20 minutes may help lower the risk of heart attack and strokes by around a third, according to a study published in *Current Biology* in 2011, but any longer than this can be counter-productive, disturbing your 24-hour circadian cycle and disrupting night-time sleep.

Work out the best time to take a nap

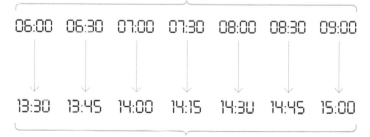

IF YOU WOKE AT

| 06:00 | 06:30 | 07:00 | 07:30 | 08:00 | 08:30 | 09:00 |

| 13:30 | 13:45 | 14:00 | 14:15 | 14:30 | 14:45 | 15:00 |

NAP TIME

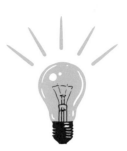

Sleep & creativity

Some of the most creative minds we know of slept very little.

Personally, I enjoy working about eighteen hours a day. Besides the short catnaps I take each day, I average about four to five hours of sleep a night.
Thomas Edison

There is some irony to the fact that the man who invented the electric light bulb, Thomas Edison, had so little regard for sleep. His creativity has had a bigger impact on sleep habits than almost anything else, allowing us to disregard the normal pattern of day and night when it comes to light.

Serious short sleepers

The artist Salvador Dali so resented spending time asleep that he devised a way to keep waking himself up. He would go to sleep holding a teaspoon in his hand, draped over the arm of a chair above a tin plate. As he dozed off and released his grip, the spoon would fall to the plate with a clatter, waking him up. Perhaps this explains the surreal, dreamlike quality of his paintings.

Sleep is the most moronic fraternity in the world, with the heaviest dues and the crudest rituals. *Vladimir Nabokov*

To sleep, perchance to dream...

Generally though, sleep deprivation doesn't suit the creative mind and the better we sleep, the more creative we are likely to be. Problem-solving, which is a feature of creativity, often occurs during slow-wave, deep sleep cycles that occur in the first four hours of sleep. REM sleep, through which we dream, also provides creative opportunities.

Paul McCartney came up with the song 'Yesterday' after dreaming its tune, while Jack Nicklaus had a dream that enabled him to correct, and improve, his golf swing. Robert Stevenson came up with the plot of the *Strange Case of Dr Jekyll and Mr Hyde* during a dream, as did Mary Shelley's *Frankenstein*. Samuel Taylor Coleridge also wrote his epic poem, 'Kubla Khan', after a dream (aided, apparently, by opium). The Periodic Table of Elements was formulated by Russian chemist Dmitri Mendeleev after sleeping on the problem, and physiologist Otto Loewi discovered in a dream the idea that allowed him to prove his theory on the chemical transmission of nerve impulses that was to win him the Nobel Prize for Medicine in 1936.

But inevitably, while the majority of studies on sleep creativity have shown that sleep can facilitate insightful behaviour and flexible reasoning, and there are several hypotheses about the creative function of dreams; there are some that support a theory of creative insomnia, in which creativity is significantly correlated with sleep disturbance.

However, for most of us, sleep is a precursor to creativity, for the simple reason that the brain functions best when it is well rested.

Man is a genius when he is sleeping

AKIRA KUROSAWA

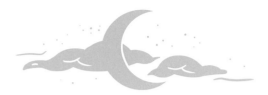

Sleep well!

> **Until you value yourself, you won't value your time.**
> **Until you value your time, you will not do anything**
> **about it.** *M. Scott Peck*

If it is your aim to sleep well, to sleep better – or, even, to sleep at all – then knowing that you have the power to change things is the first step. It may not happen immediately if your old habits are deeply entrenched, but we are geared to sleep and can return to that if we choose.

A lot of what inhibits our sleep is our attitude toward it and what we have become accustomed to. We can change our habits and we can sleep better. And we know that it will ultimately pay dividends.

In 1883, Harriet Suddoth's *The American Housekeeper's Encyclopedia*

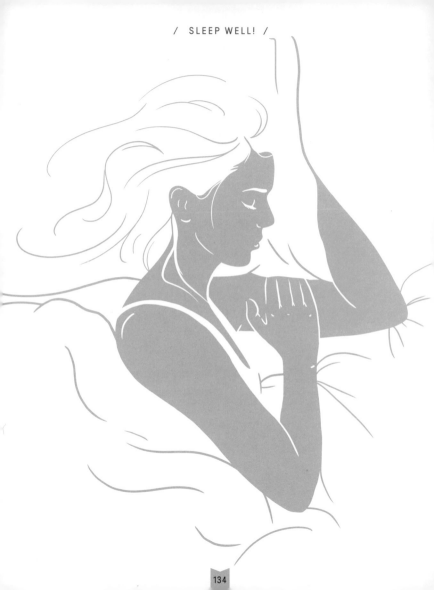

provided this solution to insomnia, designed to cool the pulse in the wrist and, by extension, the agitated heart: 'When overwakeful, get out of bed, dip a piece of cloth in water, lay this around the wrists; then wrap the dry portion over this and pin it, to keep it in place. This will exert a composing influence over the nervous system, and producing a sweet sleep, reducing the pulse; a handkerchief folded lengthwise will do. It is easy; try it.'

Today, unlike in the past, we have a far greater understanding of sleep, how it works and what can be done to both prevent it and enhance it. Knowing this means that a whole new world of restorative, restful sleep is yours to access. The rest is up to you.

Unless we begin with the right attitude, we will never find the right solution.

CHINESE PROVERB

A Better Night's Rest

Simple tips to help sleep more comfortably

SNORING/ OBSTRUCTIVE SLEEP DISORDER: Sleep on your side, rather than your back, to avoid the tongue and tissues at the falling back and impeding breathing.

NECK PAIN: Keep neck in a neutral position, with chin tucked in using only one, soft pillow above your shoulders so head is supported while keeping the pressure off the neck.

SHOULDER PAIN: Sleep on your opposite side and place a pillow beside you at chest height, over which you can drape your arm to take the pressure off the painful shoulder.

ACID REFLUX: Raise the top of the bed by placing blocks underneath, to keep stomach contents from causing reflux.

BACK PAIN:

If you sleep on your back, tuck a pillow under your knees to take the pressure off your lower spine.

If you sleep on your side, tuck a pillow between your knees, and draw them up a little to round the back.

If you sleep on your stomach, take the pressure off your lower back by tucking a pillow under your lower abdomen.

PAIN IN THE FEET: Avoid having bedclothes too heavy or tightly tucked in around the feet, which can aggravate problems like plantar fasciitis.

SLEEPING POSITIONS: 57% of people start the night sleeping on one side, while 17% sleep on their back and 11% on their stomach. The rest alternate generally between positions during the course of the night.

Acknowledgements

A huge amount of interest and body of work around the subject of sleep now exists, from which I've been able to benefit and distil the various ideas that form the basis of this book. Acknowledgement is due to the work of many sleep scientists and researchers, and in particular Professor Jim Horne and Professor Richard Wiseman.

My publisher Kate Pollard, ably assisted by Kajal Mistry, has made this the most pleasurable of publishing processes, while their talent, and that of designer Julia Murray, has contributed greatly.

Finally, in acknowledgement of my two children, Josh and Robbie: who taught me more about sleep and the lack of it than I would have previously dreamt possible!

Appendix

Further reading

Dreamland: Adventures in the strange science of sleep, David Randall, Norton & Co

I Can Make You Sleep, Paul McKenna, Bantam Press

Night School: Wake up to the power of sleep, Richard Wiseman, Macmillan

Sleepfaring: A journey through the science of sleep, Jim Horne, OUP

The Sleep Book, Dr Guy Meadows, Orion Publishing

Useful websites

www.lumie.com / www.sleepfoundation.org / www.thesleepschool.org

Apps

Sleep Cycle alarm clock / Sleepbot / Sleep Pillow
/ Relax & Sleep by Glenn Harrold / Pzizz / aSleep

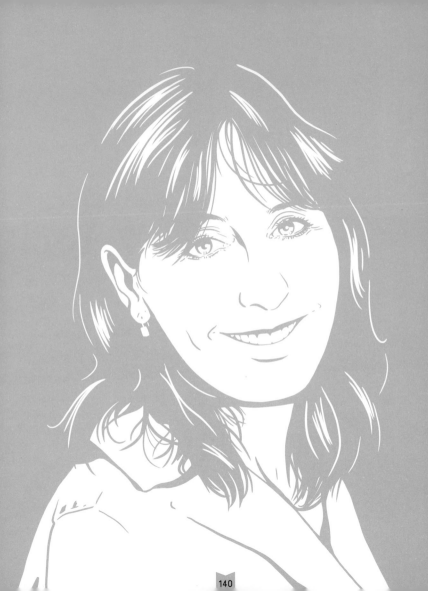

About the author

Harriet Griffey is a journalist, writer and author of numerous books focused on health. Along with *I want to sleep* she is the author of *I want to be calm* in the same series published by Hardie Grant, *The Art of Concentration*, *How to Get Pregnant* and *Give Your Child a Better Start* (with Professor Mike Howe). Harriet writes regularly on health-related and other issues for the national press. She originally trained as a nurse and is also an accredited coach with Youth at Risk (www.youthatrisk.org.uk).

Harriet

Index